Dementia

SUPPORT FOR
FAMILY AND
FRIENDS

Support for Family and Friends
Series Editors: Joanne Kerr and Alison Welsby
When a family member or friend is chronically ill or has a life-altering condition, not knowing how best to help can make you feel helpless. However, there are simple things that you can do to help both the person affected and the main carer (if this isn't you). The Support for Family and Friends series has been created for this purpose: to help you help your loved ones.

Providing up-to-date information about the illness or condition, as well as enabling you to understand what your family member or friend is going through, each book offers a wide range of ideas and advice about how to help, what to say and what to do. A useful directory of support groups and sources of information is also included so that you can access the best resources out there. You will be left feeling well informed and empowered to help – even if just to offer peace and quiet – in the most welcome and appropriate way.

Dementia

SUPPORT FOR FAMILY AND FRIENDS

Dave Pulsford and Rachel Thompson

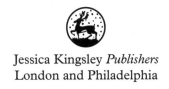

Jessica Kingsley *Publishers*
London and Philadelphia

First published in 2013
by Jessica Kingsley Publishers
73 Collier Street
London N1 9BE, UK
and
400 Market Street, Suite 400
Philadelphia, PA 19106, USA

www.jkp.com

Library of Congress Cataloging in Publication Data
Pulsford, Dave.
 Dementia : support for family and friends / Dave Pulsford and Rachel Thompson.
  p. cm.
 Includes bibliographical references and index.
 ISBN 978-1-84905-243-6 (alk. paper)
 1. Dementia--Patients--Care. 2. Dementia--Patients--Family relationships. I.
Thompson, Rachel. II. Title.
 RC521.P85 2012
 362.196'83--dc23
                                  2012016567

British Library Cataloguing in Publication Data
A CIP catalogue record for this book is available from the British Library

ISBN 978 1 84905 243 6
eISBN 978 0 85700 504 5

Printed and bound in Great Britain by Bell and Bain

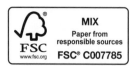

Contents

4. More Help Needed: The Phase of Moderate Dementia 103

5. The Challenges of Moderate Dementia 137

Acknowledgements

We would like to thank:

Maureen Evans, Kate Harwood, Barbara Pointon, Peter Watson and the other family members and friends of people with dementia who kindly agreed to be interviewed for this book. Thank you also to Joy Watkins at Uniting Carers, Dementia UK, for her support.

Introduction

About This Book

This book is for anyone who wants to know more about dementia and how to support those who are affected by the condition. Our readers may be close family members of someone living with dementia: their husband, wife, child or grandchild. Perhaps you have taken on or are anticipating the role of 'main carer' for the person. Alternatively you may be a close friend and want to support the person and their family. You may even have concerns about yourself. How are you feeling at this moment? We are guessing you may be feeling worried and uncertain. This is understandable; however, with guidance and support some of the fears associated with dementia can be reduced.

Whatever your relationship to the person, we hope you will find this book informative and practical in offering advice and suggestions as to how to make the life of someone with dementia as pleasant and fulfilled as possible, while also supporting yourselves and each other. Above all, we hope that we can assist you to take on a positive attitude towards living with dementia. For although being a family member or a friend of a person with dementia can be difficult, wearying and sometimes heart-breaking, with your help and that of others, including paid carers and professionals, the person can have a good quality of life and experience a sense of well-being right up to the end of their life. This means that you can take some comfort and satisfaction in knowing that you have done your best for the person and those close to them.

Dementia is a progressive and terminal condition for which there is as yet no cure. However, there is much that can be done to help people who have it. We assume in this book that our readers are committed to making life for a person with dementia the best it can be, but need knowledge, understanding and skills in order to do so. Important aspects of knowledge include information about the type of dementia the person has, how dementia will affect the person and others, and what sources of outside or professional support are available.

Understanding is needed of how people with dementia experience the condition; what their feelings are likely to be; and, importantly, how they experience the world through the cognitive difficulties that are the main feature of dementia. We call this 'dementia empathy' and regard this quality as the most important factor in successfully supporting a person with dementia. We will discuss this concept in some depth throughout the book. Important skills include being able to communicate effectively with someone with dementia, helping the person keep active and independent, and responding effectively if the person behaves in ways that others may find difficult.

Also, the journey through dementia will include many decision-making points, where either the person themselves or those close to them must decide on future courses of action. We believe the information and ideas in this book will assist our readers with decision making and, where possible, encourage them to include the person with dementia in reaching decisions. The content derives from our experience as practitioners, teachers and researchers in the field of dementia care. We also bring in the voices of family members and friends of people with dementia by including quotes from interviewees who have very kindly offered their own experiences of caring for and supporting someone with dementia.

Dementia is a progressive condition that may take years to reach its conclusion. The person is likely to pass through broadly defined phases on their journey through dementia, although each person may have slightly different symptoms. These phases have been termed early (or mild), moderate, and advanced (or severe) dementia. We have adopted the approach of structuring this book to reflect the progressive nature of dementia and, although there will be some individual variations in how dementia progresses, we hope it offers a useful framework. We begin in Chapter 1 with a broad overview of dementia, general information about its nature, and the fundamental principles of caring for and supporting a person with dementia. Chapter 2 discusses how dementia may begin and the process of assessment that can lead to a diagnosis. We also consider some of the specific types of dementia. In Chapter 3 we focus on the early phase of dementia, when a person retains many of their abilities and the main role of family members and friends is to help the person retain independence while planning for the future. In Chapter 4 we address the phase of moderate dementia, in which a person requires more active care and support and their difficulties mean that maintaining independence may be problematic. As the phase of moderate dementia leads to the most profound changes in the person and often the greatest challenges for family members and friends, we continue to consider that phase in Chapter 5. In Chapter 6 we discuss the issues surrounding long-term residential care: whether or not to seek a residential care place for the person, how to choose a care home and how to support the person living in a care home. Chapter 7 addresses the phase of advanced dementia, in which the person's difficulties are such that they require more or less complete care from others, whether family members and friends or professionals. Finally, as dementia is inevitably a terminal condition, we contemplate the end of life in Chapter 8. Specific issues will be discussed within the book at the point in the journey through dementia that they are most likely to arise, but it must always be remembered that people with dementia are all individuals and the condition may progress and affect people in different ways.

Our focus is on general principles of care and support that can be applied to people with dementia worldwide. Most English-speaking countries have broadly similar professional care services and underpinning legal frameworks for people with dementia, but there are inevitably differences in a number of areas. These include support service provision, funding arrangements, legislation and sometimes terminology. We do not attempt to discuss specifics such as the structure of care services, funding arrangements or legal frameworks in different countries, but we include a 'Resources for Family and Friends' section at the end of the book that details specific resources and other sources of support for those living in the UK, the USA, Australia and elsewhere.

'Understanding more about dementia and knowing what to expect has helped me know how to respond and cope better.'

CHAPTER I

Becoming Acquainted with Dementia

What is dementia?

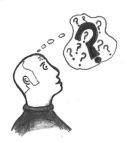

Dementia is a condition that results from disease of the brain. In medical terms, dementia is a *syndrome* – that is to say, a set of difficulties that a person experiences that can result from a number of underlying causes. Over a hundred different types of dementia have been identified – fortunately the majority of them are extremely uncommon. In most cases dementia does not affect a person until later in life – the large majority of people with dementia are 65 or older – but some diseases that lead to dementia can affect younger people. The most common types of dementia are Alzheimer's disease, vascular dementia, dementia with Lewy bodies and fronto-temporal dementia. We will describe these and other forms of dementia in the next chapter.

People can live with dementia for a long time, so supporting their quality of life is essential. It is important though to recognise that dementia is a progressive and terminal condition that will in most cases lead to increasing cognitive difficulties and dependence on others. How long a person will live depends upon the type of dementia, their age and their general health, but many will live with the condition for several years. Eventually though, a person with dementia is likely to die as a result of the condition, although some may develop other illnesses that can lead to death, such as heart disease or cancer, particularly if the person is older. This of course makes dementia particularly difficult for family members and friends. They have the pain of seeing someone they know and love deteriorate and change, and they also need to come to terms early on with the probability of eventually losing that person. It also means that it is important to think about and plan for the future and, although this can be hard to face, it is an issue that needs addressing (see Chapter 3).

People with dementia are not all the same, and individuals will have their own particular difficulties. There are a number of reasons for this. First, as stated earlier, there are many types of dementia, and each may have different features, especially in the early phase. Second, because dementia is a progressive condition, some features are more obvious in the earlier phase while others appear more in the later phases. Third, factors in a person's make-up, such as their personality, life history, and physical and mental health, will influence how dementia is manifested. Finally, the way a person is interacted with and cared for by family members, friends and professionals can have a big effect on how dementia progresses. We will consider these factors in more detail in subsequent chapters. Overall, however, the following are the main difficulties that arise as a result of dementia.

MEMORY DIFFICULTIES

Often, but not always, these are the first signs of dementia. A person may begin to forget things that they would normally have no trouble remembering. Initially, these are likely to be memories of recent events, or newly learnt information. The person might forget someone's name, or what they did the previous day. They might say something as part of a conversation, and then soon after say it again, forgetting that they have already done so. If they are told something new, they might not remember it, or they might find it hard to keep up with what is going on around them. The important thing is that this is a *change* from the way the person is usually – all of us have memory lapses from time to time, and memory difficulties are only a sign of dementia if the person's memory seems worse than it used to be and other changes are also apparent.

> 'It was particularly my husband's memory; he was continually asking me what the time was, what date it was, what we were going to be doing. He previously would have been more in control.'

As dementia progresses, memory difficulties are likely to worsen. In the early phase of dementia, a person is still able to remember very familiar information, such as the names of close family members, or where to find things in the home. Also, the person can remember events from the past, often back as far as childhood. As time goes on, however, these memories become damaged and eventually lost as well, and in the advanced phase of dementia the person may appear to have little memory for either new or past events, and live their life entirely in the present moment.

CHANGES IN MANNER AND EMOTIONS

The first sign of some types of dementia may not be memory loss but apparent changes in personality – a person's manner or outlook on life. Some people may seem to be more inclined to touchiness or anger than is usual for them, while others may seem quieter and more subdued, or more anxious about events. These signs may not be recognised for what they are, and family members and friends of the person may think that they are depressed or under stress. This can often happen with younger people who have dementia (those aged 65 or below), because changes in manner and behaviour are common first signs of some of the conditions that affect these age groups.

Such changes may become more noticeable as dementia progresses, and may be reflected in a person behaving in ways that others find difficult, such as becoming very agitated or perhaps resistive and even aggressive in certain situations. Some individuals can become very emotional and cry or become upset much more than they used to. Others may become apathetic and disinclined to do things, and may well suffer from depression. Individuals are very variable, however, and some people may show few changes in their manner or in their usual mood.

'Grandad would describe Grandma as being quite stubborn and awkward and those were things that I just couldn't picture in her.'

'My husband had begun to be very impatient with my mother and he was normally very patient and kind. He started shouting at her – very out of character.'

DECLINE IN COGNITIVE ABILITIES

'Cogntive' relates to a person's intellectual or thinking abilities. Dementia affects people's cognitive abilities in many ways. Family and friends will notice them finding it harder to do many things that they used to be able to do. The person's general thinking abilities will decline – if, for example, they used to be good at crosswords or maths problems or pub quizzes, they may find them increasingly difficult. The person's attention span may reduce, and they may progressively find it harder to concentrate on things for more than a brief period of time, or to attend to things outside their immediate field of view. Their judgement may be affected and they may find it harder to make decisions, or be unable to take account of all the factors involved in decision making. This may lead to them sometimes wanting to do things that might risk harm to themselves or others. One example of this is when a person believes that they are still able to drive a car without any problems, when in fact they are at risk of getting lost or having an accident.

What can also decline is a person's ability to carry out tasks that involve a sequence of actions, such as getting dressed or making a cup of tea (psychologists call this 'impairment of executive function'). The person may put their clothes on in the wrong order, or be unable to button their shirt. Ultimately this can lead to people losing the ability to look after themselves and needing help with eating and drinking, keeping themselves clean and managing their continence needs.

> 'I was teaching my wife how to play dominoes and she had no clue that you had to match the numbers together. I thought that was really strange. One day my wife found she couldn't make sandwiches. She was just stood there with two pieces of ham and four pieces of bread, not knowing what to do.'

It is not unusual for individuals to try and cover up any difficulties they are experiencing, particularly in the early phase, and it may take a while for families and friends to recognise changes. Often a person will make excuses in order to avoid taking on tasks or finding themselves in situations where they feel exposed.

> 'I could see that my husband's confidence was ebbing away. He even came to me one day as he couldn't work out how to wire a 3-pin plug properly; this was a man who used to construct electronic equipment from scratch.'

> 'My husband wasn't doing as much as he used to; we always had a very equal relationship but he was beginning to do less. He'd say things like "your cooking is better than mine" – I accepted it at the time but when I look back I think it was an excuse.'

Yet another effect of memory and cognitive difficulties is *disorientation*. This is where a person has problems knowing where they are or finding their way about, understanding the concept of time, or being able to recognise other people. Disorientation tends to become more pronounced as the condition progresses and eventually the person appears to lack understanding of the world around them.

'I think one of the first things I noticed was when we were on holiday staying in a hotel and my wife couldn't find her way back to the room. I did think it was a bit odd but I didn't really think much about it at the time... I just thought she was being stupid.'

With some types of dementia, difficulties can be encountered with such matters as visual or spatial perception – the ability to follow things visually or to understand how things relate to each other in the physical world.

'My husband started to make mistakes in his piano playing – it felt to him as if his right hand and the left hand weren't getting their acts together. He was absolutely frustrated, he kept practising and practising to re-teach his hands but in fact what was happening was his eye travelling from one line of music to the next that was the problem.'

BEHAVIOUR CHANGES

It will be apparent that a person's memory, manner and cognitive difficulties are likely to lead to considerable changes in the ways that the person behaves and acts. We have mentioned that the person will find some abilities declining, leading them to do less than they did before. The person may also start to behave in different ways and to do things that may be hard for others to understand, such as hiding away or hoarding things or having a strong need to walk about. Sometimes the person may behave in ways that families and friends find very difficult, such as being extremely irritable or agitated. Such behaviour may often seem random and inexplicable, but as we will see in Chapter 5 it may well have meaning for the person.

'I thought my husband was doing it deliberately; he used to take my oven gloves and throw them on top of the kitchen cabinet where I couldn't get them. Instead he was hiding them safely because he knew they were important and shouldn't get lost. I thought he was being difficult.'

COMMUNICATION DIFFICULTIES

The impairment of memory and cognition that comes with dementia often shows itself by a person having problems communicating with and understanding others. In the early phase of dementia, the person can usually understand what others are saying, but may find it hard to express themselves in a clear way. Initially, the person's difficulty might be in finding the right name for something (including very familiar words such as 'dog' or 'coat'). Later, the person may find it hard to put together sentences that are understandable to others, even though they know what they want to say (the term that psychologists use for this is 'expressive dysphasia'). This is obviously very frustrating for the person and hard for those family members and friends with whom the person is trying to communicate.

> 'One time Mum couldn't get words out and she got upset and she lashed out at me. It was as though she wanted to tear her hair out, she was in such a state and I had to hold her hands and say, "Don't do that to me Mum, I'm only trying to help you. I hate what's happening to you." And she ended up getting upset and I got upset too.'

Sometimes, what a person says reflects disordered ways of thinking. They may develop a firm belief that something is true when it really isn't. This may mean that they are misinterpreting things or it could be what psychologists call 'delusional thinking'. Sometimes this can cause distress for the person and their family and friends, such as when the person firmly believes that others are stealing things from them, or that their mother is alive and coming to visit, when in fact she died many years ago. It is important to understand that in many cases this kind of thinking is a result of people trying to make sense of the world around them in the context of their fading memory and thinking abilities, and creating a reality that helps them to cope.

Other people may hear voices in their heads or see things that aren't actually there ('auditory or visual hallucinations'), and talk as if they were real. In some types of dementia this can be a significant feature. It is also not uncommon for older people to experience problems with their eyesight, which if not corrected can lead to visual misperceptions. It is important to establish the cause and recognise that these experiences are part of the condition. We will discuss how to respond to such communication issues in Chapter 4.

A common difficulty experienced in communication is that people with dementia become repetitive: they may ask the same questions again and again, or utter the same phrases many times over. Much of the time this occurs as a result of memory loss and the person will have simply forgotten they have said something a few minutes before.

> 'The first sign was that Grandma would repeat herself, ask the same question again or say the same thing over and over again.'

As the condition progresses to the phase of advanced dementia, a person may seem to lose the ability to understand what others are saying to them – we say 'seem to' because by this point the person may have lost the ability to talk meaningfully to other people and so we can't really tell if they can understand us or not. It may well be that the person still understands something of what we are saying to them – it is likely they will pick up on the feelings behind the words that we are uttering and be comforted or distressed according to what those feelings are. Again, we will say more about how to communicate effectively with people with advanced dementia in Chapter 7.

PHYSICAL PROBLEMS

As we have discussed earlier, dementia is a progressive condition and in the later phase a person may experience noticeable physical decline. There are a number of physical changes that may develop as the illness progresses, including problems with eating, drinking, using the toilet and walking. In addition to this, some types of dementia have physical symptoms throughout their course as well as the psychological symptoms that we have been describing (see Chapter 2).

REDUCED AWARENESS

'Awareness' refers to the extent that a person with dementia is aware that they have the condition, and understands the effects that dementia is having on them. People vary in how aware they are. In the early phase of dementia, some people have considerable awareness of their condition and its implications. This allows them both to take action to compensate for their difficulties, and to make plans for the future when their level of awareness will be reduced. With others, awareness declines from the outset and the person may deny that there is anything wrong with them. This of course can create problems for family members and friends because the person may not accept their help, or may insist on carrying on with activities that they are no longer able to perform safely.

As dementia progresses, awareness tends to decline along with a person's cognitive ability, and the person may lack understanding of why others are not letting them do certain things, such as going out of the house on their own, or are apparently insisting on doing things to them, such as making them have a wash or go to the toilet.

The extent of dementia worldwide

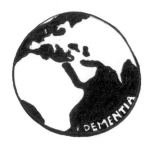

While dementia can affect people at any age, it is by far most common in older people and the longer one lives the greater the chance one has of developing it. Life expectancy is increasing in most countries and that means that there are many more people with dementia worldwide than there used to be. A report published in 2009 by the organization Alzheimer's Disease International estimated that 36 million people worldwide are living with dementia, and that numbers are expected to double every 20 years (Prince and Jackson 2009).

Few families have been unaffected by dementia and it may be helpful for readers to know that they are far from alone in having to come to terms with it. A recent study estimates that there are at present around 820,000 people with dementia in the UK (Luengo-Fernandez, Leal and Gray 2010), while the Alzheimer's Association's latest figures suggest that there are 5.4 million people with dementia in the USA (Alzheimer's Association 2012). At the same time, dementia is not just an issue for industrialised societies; despite generally lower life expectancy, the large majority of people with dementia live in developing countries with much of the expected increase in numbers being in low- and middle-income countries. This is obviously significant in financial terms with the worldwide costs of dementia, according to the *World Alzheimer Report*, being estimated as US$604 billion in 2010, amounting to more than 1 per cent of global domestic product (Price and Jackson 2009). It is said that, if dementia care were a country, it would be the world's 18th largest economy.

Dementia is not, however, an inevitable consequence of growing older. Fewer than 10 per cent of those below the age of 80 will have dementia, and less than a quarter in their 80s will be affected (Knapp and Prince 2007). It will not comfort those with dementia in their family to know that they are in a minority, but there is no inevitability that even if we live to 100 that we will develop dementia – less than two-fifths of centenarians have the condition.

Dementia in 'minority groups'

Dementia can potentially affect everyone but it is important to consider the particular issues and needs of those groups that do not make up the majority of people with dementia.

YOUNG-ONSET DEMENTIA

As has been seen, the majority of cases of dementia are classed as 'late onset', defined as dementia that manifests itself when a person is over the age of 65. Dementia can, however, affect people at any age and a proportion of people will have young-onset dementia. This is sometimes also called 'early-onset' or 'working-age' dementia and is when the signs of dementia appear before the person has reached 65. In the UK, around 17,000 people have a diagnosis of young-onset dementia and in the USA around 200,000 have been diagnosed. These figures are likely to be underestimates, as a result of misdiagnosis of symptoms (Prince and Jackson 2009).

Sometimes the disease process is the same as for late-onset dementia, but often different diseases with their own particular features lead to young-onset dementia – we will overview some of the more common conditions in the next chapter. Young-onset dementia carries its own particular challenges for a person, their family, friends and professionals. They have more to give up – they are more likely to have a job and they may have child-rearing and financial responsibilities that will have to be taken on by other family members while they are also caring for the person with dementia. A younger person with dementia may be more physically fit and active, which means that it can be harder to meet their needs for activity and can lead to more acute problems if the person's behaviour causes difficulties to others. Also, the rarity of young-onset dementia can lead to issues with providing professional support services or residential care; because there will be comparatively few people with young-onset dementia in a particular geographical area, it can be hard to provide specific services and younger people may be forced into services designed for older adults because of a lack of more appropriate alternatives. This can be compounded by the fact that different forms of young-onset dementia have very different features from each other, leading to experts suggesting that services for younger people should be specific to the type of dementia – even harder to provide for small numbers of people.

ETHNIC MINORITY AND IMMIGRANT GROUPS AND DEMENTIA

Some countries have small but growing immigrant groups whose cultural beliefs about and approach to dementia may be different from those of the majority culture. People from some cultures might not think of dementia as a disease process. For example, it is a fact that in some South Asian languages there is no word for dementia, because the cognitive processes that lead to dementia are regarded simply as an aspect of ageing that will eventually happen to everyone to a lesser or greater extent.

It is also well established that some minority groups use professional support services and especially residential care to a much lesser extent than the majority population. This can lead professionals to the belief that they have no need to work with people with dementia and their families from some minority ethnic groups as 'the family looks after their own'. The reality is rather more complex. Certainly, some groups, such as those from South Asian and Chinese cultures, have traditional values that families should take responsibility for older or needy members. But there is also sometimes a feeling that professional services may not be able to meet their needs because of a lack of cultural understanding. It is also the case that family carers from minority ethnic groups can experience as much stress and burden as those from the majority population and so could benefit as much from outside help. A further factor is the cultural changes that are occurring as immigrant groups become settled in their adopted country and some of their children take on more 'Westernised' values, with perhaps less of a sense of family obligation.

It may also be the case that some types of dementia are more prevalent in some racial groups. For example, recent research has indicated that Afro-Americans or people from Afro-Caribbean backgrounds in the UK may be more likely to develop dementia (Adelman *et al.* 2011; Alzheimer's Association 2002).

PEOPLE WITH LEARNING DISABILITIES AND DEMENTIA

There are strong links between learning disabilities such as Down's syndrome and dementia. People with learning disabilities are at higher risk of developing dementia, and tend to develop it at an earlier age than the population as a whole. In the past this was less of an issue because people with learning disabilities tended to have relatively low life expectancy. Today, medical advances and improved social care have lengthened life expectancy for people with learning disabilities, leading to growing numbers with dementia. It might be thought that dementia is not so problematic for a person with learning disabilities because they are already cognitively disabled. However, dementia can lead to profound negative changes in a person's cognitive abilities, which can result in the person becoming more disabled than before and cause as much distress to the person's family and friends as with anyone else who develops dementia. It can also, as with others, shorten the person's life expectancy.

GAY, LESBIAN, BISEXUAL AND TRANSGENDERED PEOPLE WITH DEMENTIA

Readers who are a family member, partner or friend of a gay, lesbian, bisexual or transgendered (GLBT) person who develops dementia will of course face the same issues as anyone else. However, in some ways the experience of GLBT people with dementia can be different from the experience of those who are heterosexual, particularly when it comes to interacting with professionals who may lack understanding of their needs or even awareness of their situation. GLBT people may be more likely to become detached from their families, leading to fewer sources of support if they develop dementia. They may have hidden their sexuality for years and they and their partners may not feel able to be open with professionals about the true nature of their relationship, which can lead to the needs and potential contributions of their partners being ignored by professionals. Some who have worked in residential care have had the experience of a resident being visited regularly by a 'close friend' of the same sex without realising that the friend was the resident's partner – or thinking to ask the visitor if that was the case.

FAMILIES AND FRIENDS OF 'MINORITY GROUP' MEMBERS WITH DEMENTIA

If you are a family member or friend of a person with dementia who fits into one of these 'minority groups', you may recognise some of the extra challenges that this implies. We will discuss specific issues relevant to these groups as this book progresses. However, the goals of dementia care and the principles of supporting a person with dementia are the same regardless of the person's circumstances. Quality of life and well-being are still paramount, and understanding how to assist the person to attain these goals is key to supporting them in their journey through dementia.

Can dementia be treated, cured or prevented?

Our first thought on hearing that someone we are close to has an illness is can it be treated or cured? The blunt answer to this question as far as dementia is concerned is that with our current state of understanding there is no cure for any type of dementia, although researchers offer hope that this situation may change. There are some drugs that offer short-term relief of symptoms for Alzheimer's disease and new drugs that may further delay the progression of dementia are being trialled. We will discuss these in the next chapter.

PREVENTING DEMENTIA

There is growing evidence that aspects of our lifestyle may influence whether or not we will develop dementia and may perhaps influence the progression of the condition. As we will see in the next chapter, there is clear evidence that cardiovascular factors are present in the most common types of dementia that affect people in later life, and a lifestyle that may protect against cardiovascular diseases, such as hypertension (high blood pressure), diabetes, heart attack and stroke, may also protect against dementia. Simple health behaviours such as avoiding smoking, drinking alcohol within safe limits, maintaining recommended body weight and eating a 'Mediterranean' diet minimising red meat and saturated fat and including plenty of fruit and vegetables and oily fish, are as relevant to preventing dementia as they are to warding off other illnesses. Maintaining regular exercise into old age is also important, with strong research evidence that moderate exercise done on a regular basis may reduce the risk of dementia.

Another factor that appears to influence dementia is educational engagement, and in particular maintaining intelligence-based activity into old age. If we continue as we grow older to carry out mind-stimulating activities such as reading, crosswords and puzzles, learning new things and playing musical instruments, we may delay the onset of dementia or at least keep our brains active and stimulated enough to help slow deterioration. However, one should be wary of 'brain-training' books or computer packages that advertise their ability to ward off dementia. None has a firm evidence base and keeping up a generally social and mentally stimulating lifestyle into old age is likely to have a greater protective effect than once in a while carrying out specific brain-training exercises.

In short, there are things we can do to reduce our own risk of developing dementia and there is evidence that treating cardiovascular factors such as high blood pressure and high cholesterol, helping a person remain physically active and promoting cognitive stimulation may help slow the progression of dementia in those who have the condition. While there is still much to be learnt about dementia and we are many years away from eradicating it, we are not completely helpless in protecting ourselves and those people with dementia who are our family members and friends from the worst effects of the condition.

The goals of supporting a person with dementia: quality of life and well-being

We mentioned in the introduction to this book that, by family members and friends supporting a person with dementia, that person may achieve the best quality of life possible, and experience as much as possible a sense of well-being. What do these concepts really mean, and how can family members and friends help a person with dementia reach these goals?

'Quality of life' and 'well-being' are rather vague concepts, but ones that we can apply to ourselves. We could all make a list of those things that we feel enhance our quality of life and make us feel good – folk music concerts, red wine, reading, swimming, country walks and meals out with families and friends feature highly on our own lists! In the early phase of dementia, when people still retain many of their abilities, there is no reason why their lives cannot broadly continue as before so that to an extent at least they can derive well-being from their accustomed activities and pastimes. As a person's range of abilities starts to narrow, however, some preferred activities may on the face of it become difficult or perhaps seem impossible. At the same time, a person with dementia will derive well-being from the same broad aspects of experience as we all do.

RECEIVING AFFECTION, DIGNITY AND RESPECT

We will all undoubtedly agree that these are important to our own sense of well-being. It can take as little as an aggressive driver sounding his horn at us unnecessarily to put a cloud on our day, and arguments and ill-feeling within the family will of course make us feel bad. People who have dementia are no different. As dementia progresses, the ways that family members and friends interact with the person are put into sharper perspective, with little things that others say and do having a strong influence on the person's sense of well-being or ill-being (see Chapter 4).

KEEPING ACTIVE

Many people with dementia will have been active throughout their lives and will have a need to keep active as dementia progresses. This may simply take the form of wanting to be on their feet and walking about, or it may at some level reflect the desire to continue leisure or work activities that they once enjoyed. Of course, many activities also involve socialising with others. One of the strongest contributions that family members and friends can make to enhance the well-being of people with dementia is to help them keep active, either by assisting them to keep up pastimes that they previously enjoyed or by finding new things that they can do despite their difficulties. Above all, people want to feel included and involved at whatever stage they are at, and the more we can do to enable this the better it will be for the person. Indeed people in the early stage of dementia are now beginning to speak out and say, 'I am living with dementia, not dying from it.'

MAINTAINING INDEPENDENCE

Many people with physical difficulties have a strong need to maintain independence and to do things for themselves rather than have others do things for them. Those with cognitive difficulties such as dementia are the same. This may in the early phase of dementia be reflected in a desire to continue to live independently and giving up that independence can be difficult. In the later phases of dementia, maintaining independence is linked to keeping active: the more people can do for themselves, whether it is helping around the house, pursuing hobbies or simply getting themselves washed and dressed, the more they are maintaining a level of activity. Also such activity, requiring an element of thinking for themselves, helps provide cognitive stimulation, which as seen earlier may help slow the progression of dementia. It may be that people will need supervision or indeed get things 'wrong' but the opportunity to stay involved is vital.

> 'My grandma will walk over to the supermarket every day to get the things she needs…that's her pleasure, that's the only thing she does. If we take away going to the supermarket from her, she'd have no quality of life.'

MAKING CHOICES

Independence and choice making are of course strongly linked: being independent implies choosing how to live our lives. In the early phase of dementia, the person is likely to retain considerable capacity for making choices about their life. However, there may be times when reduced awareness or insight may result in their making choices that are not in their best interests, such as refusing help or wanting to continue activities that put themselves at risk. In these situations, the role of family and friends in supporting the right choice is extremely important and can require great skill and diplomacy. As well as helping the person make choices in the present, family members and friends can assist them to make choices about their future, through drawing up 'living wills' or 'advance decisions' regarding what they would want to happen when they cannot make important decisions for themselves (discussed in Chapter 3).

In the later phases of dementia, major decision making may be very difficult for a person, but offering choices should not be ruled out altogether. It will enhance dignity and respect for the person if we ask them what their choice would be where possible rather than deciding for them, even if it as simple a matter as 'Would you like tea or coffee?'

EXPERIENCING FAMILIARITY AND CONTINUITY

People with dementia will often feel more secure and content in an environment that is familiar and with a routine that maintains continuity and minimises major changes. This is partly because more longstanding memories are retained better than recent memories, so the person may recognise things and people that remind them of long-term aspects of their life and derive comfort from that recognition. Also, while people with dementia can adapt to new environments and learn new things, too much change and unfamiliarity will be hard for them to take in and come to terms with. Family members and friends will of course assist a person with dementia to experience familiarity simply by their presence as people that the person knows and loves. They can also contribute to promoting a familiar environment for the person even if they have to move to residential care, by passing on their knowledge of the person and their life to care staff, or by making the person's living area more like home by bringing in some of their possessions or photographs.

RECEIVING HELP WHERE NEEDED

While these principles are noble ones, it will be evident that as dementia progresses a person will need more and more assistance from others with managing their lives as their range of abilities narrows. As time goes on the balance between promoting independence and doing things that the person cannot do for themselves will shift. At every phase, the person will need a level of help to compensate for their cognitive difficulties. Ultimately this may include providing assistance with basic needs such as eating, drinking and keeping clean. To what extent this help will come from families and friends or from professional carers will depend on a range of factors, but at every phase of dementia, and whether or not the person is receiving full-time professional care, family members and friends will have a role to play in helping to ensure that the person's needs are met.

Being a family member or friend of a person with dementia

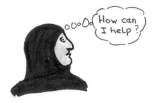

Given that dementia is a long-term progressive condition that will lead sooner or later to cognitive decline and dependence, how should we regard dementia and what should be our role as family members and friends? This is a difficult question but one that has considerable implications for our relationship with the person with dementia and for their own future. It will be evident that, because of the nature of their difficulties, people with dementia can become particularly reliant on others, not just to ensure their safety and physical health, but for their sense of well-being also. And that means they rely on family and friends.

How do we feel about being in this crucial but demanding position? Our natural reaction to dementia may be a negative one. We may be filled with foreboding when we think of the journey ahead and the emotional and physical demands it may impose on us. We may experience a gradual and continuing sense of loss as the person we knew starts to drift away, to be replaced by a very different kind of person who may bear little resemblance to our loved one. This sense of loss may make us want to distance ourselves from the person. This attitude was succinctly expressed by an acquaintance who said that she was reluctant to visit her grandmother with dementia because 'it isn't really her'. Alternatively, for some it may be an opportunity to become closer through having a new role of providing support and care.

As a person's understanding of the world diminishes, the familiarity of family and friends becomes more and more important to them. Even in the advanced phase of dementia, when the person may not recognise those closest to them, the emotional comfort that only the presence of a loved one can provide will help them experience a measure of well-being. This is not to suggest that families and friends should be morally obliged to take on all the work of caring for a person with dementia. Caring for a friend or family member who has dementia can be very stressful, particularly when behaviour changes, and it is not a role everyone feels they can take on. It is possible for professional carers who have the right understanding and skills to provide much needed emotional comfort and support. Professional help is vital at all phases of the journey through dementia and, as we will discuss in Chapter 6, residential care may eventually be the most appropriate option for some people with dementia. Family members or friends can sometimes feel guilty of having failed in some way if they hand over direct care. But even if the person goes to live in a care home, the contributions of families and friends should not be underestimated.

BECOMING A MAIN CARER

It will be evident from what has been said previously that supporting a person with dementia places considerable responsibility on families and friends and is a responsibility that some will feel better able to take on than others. Many people with dementia of course want to live in the community in familiar surroundings and with familiar people, and many families want that for them as well. We have seen earlier how independence, familiarity and continuity, and the presence of loved ones, will enhance the quality of life of a person with dementia.

It is typical with people with dementia living in the community that a particular person, usually a close family member, sometimes a friend, takes on the role of main carer. That person does most of the work of caring, becomes the person that the individual with dementia most relates to and is the one who liaises with professional services. Sometimes the main carer takes on the role voluntarily and would prefer that they had that role rather than other family members. Sometimes, however, a person can become the main carer by default, because they are the person's only relative, or other family members are unable or unwilling to take on the responsibility and subtly (sometimes unsubtly) push another into the caring role. In such circumstances, it is not surprising to learn that women are more likely to take on the role of main carer to a person with dementia than men. Such family dynamics are perhaps inevitable but clearly place the bulk of the caring responsibility onto one person, who may feel unsupported or abandoned if other family members or friends then step back and leave them to it. It should be the responsibility of family members and friends that the main carer is not abandoned in this way.

The basis of supporting a person with dementia: dementia empathy

Whether one is a person's main carer, a family member or a friend, understanding is needed of how to support or care for the person with dementia. We base our approach on one basic principle: that family members and friends should attempt to empathise with the person, by trying to appreciate how they are feeling and also, importantly, how they understand the world around them through the screen that their cognitive difficulties place between them and their world. We call this 'dementia empathy' – empathising with the person's cognitive difficulties. If we can achieve this, we can help the person in more than one way. First, we can assist the person to manage their life by finding ways of compensating for their cognitive difficulties, just as we help people who have physical difficulties. Second, by recognising that the person's actions or words reflect their cognitive difficulties, we can avoid blaming the person when they do or say things that we may find frustrating or upsetting – we can with honesty say to ourselves that 'they can't help it' and seek to find ways of reducing such misunderstandings or minimising their effects on others.

DEMENTIA EMPATHY, COGNITIVE DIFFICULTIES AND 'CONFUSION'

The cognitive difficulties that people with dementia develop may affect their ability to manage their lives in two broad ways. First, they may *misunderstand* the world around them, including other people. If a family member or friend says something to a person, they may misinterpret it, or just not understand it at all. They may not recognise who is talking to them, even if it is a close family member or friend. Similarly, they may misinterpret aspects of their environment, such as reading the weather wrong or failing to recognise where they are. For some people there can be visual-spatial difficulties – problems with judging distances or interpreting visual signs or cues. It is also possible for someone to develop false perceptions or hallucinations (seeing or hearing things that are not really there and responding to them as if they were real), or false beliefs or delusions (believing something to be real and responding accordingly).

The second way that people with dementia may experience cognitive difficulties is through reduced ability to *respond* to the world around them. A person may understand what has been said to them but may not be able to find the right words to answer. They may know where they are but be unsure how to get to where they want to go. They may see and recognise a cup, kettle and packet of tea bags on the kitchen shelf but be unable to work out how to make a cup of tea. If asked to decide on something, they may understand the issues but lack the ability to put those issues together to make a decision. Figure 1.1 summarises the main cognitive difficulties that dementia can cause, divided into these two broad categories.

Put together, these difficulties lead to a person displaying what we commonly term 'confusion'. Confusion is a blanket term for behaviour, speech or manner that comes from the person either misunderstanding the world around them, or not being able to respond appropriately to the world around them, or both. It is important for family members and friends to look beyond the rather stark term 'confusion' and try to identify the specific difficulties that the person has with relating to the world.

Understanding the basis of a person's cognitive difficulties is the key to dementia empathy. If we can, as it were, get inside the head of the person with dementia and appreciate how they perceive the world around them, and if we can recognise when the person can respond appropriately to events in the world and when they can't, we can then come up with ways of helping them compensate for their difficulties. Throughout this book we will refer to the concept of dementia empathy when interpreting aspects of a person with dementia's behaviour or offering advice and tips as to how we might help the person live their life more effectively.

Difficulties with understanding the world

Failing to recognise a person who is talking to them

Misunderstanding what a person is saying to them

Failing to recognise where they are

Failing to recognise familiar objects

Misinterpreting visual cues

Experiencing false perceptions (auditory or visual hallucinations)

Experiencing false beliefs (delusions)

Difficulty in paying attention to what is happening around them

Difficulty with taking in or remembering information

Thinking they are in another place or a different time in their life

Difficulties with responding to the world

Forgetting to do things they need to do

Knowing what they want to say but not finding the right words

Responding to misperceptions, hallucinations and delusions rather than to the 'real' world

Having difficulty in carrying out tasks in the right order

Knowing where they are but not how to get to where they need to go

Difficulty with weighing up information

Difficulty with making appropriate decisions

Difficulty with getting their needs met in an appropriate way

FIGURE 1.1 THE COGNITIVE DIFFICULTIES OF DEMENTIA

SUPPORTING THE PERSON: ASSISTANCE VERSUS INDEPENDENCE

When helping a person with dementia compensate for their cognitive difficulties, family members and friends sometimes have a difficult balancing act to perform. On the one hand, we want to ensure that the person gets their needs met quickly and appropriately. On the other hand, we should be aiming for the person to be as independent as possible. As we have seen, independence carries lots of benefits for a person with dementia: it helps keep them active, it enhances well-being and it may even slow the progression of dementia. This means that family and friends should be trying to assist the person with dementia to do things for themselves and only to do things for the person if it is clear that they are unable to do those things unaided.

A simple analogy can be made with physical disability. Suppose a person has weakness in their legs and finds it hard to stand up out of a chair. If we see the person struggling to rise, we are tempted to go over and help them up. Our motivation for doing so is often twofold: first, we want to make things easier and less effort for the person and, second, we want to reduce the risk of the person falling and coming to harm. The same motives lie behind our wanting to do things for a person with dementia. Often it can seem easier to do something for the person, whether it is tidying their house, making them a cup of tea or, in the later phases, getting them dressed, rather than watch them slowly struggle to do it themselves. Also, we sometimes see genuine risks in the person being independent, of their accidentally coming to harm, or even being exploited and abused by others. Balancing the risks of independence with the benefits is one of the hardest tasks for those supporting a person with dementia, and deciding when to intervene and take away an aspect of independence can be very difficult, especially if the person believes they can still be independent in that aspect. We will explore such situations as we go through this book.

'My husband's very restless and wants to go out and walk around all the time. I used to do this with him but I've accepted

I can't go with him all the time now so have to "take the risk" and hope that he'll be safe. But as he gets more confused about the time of day I expect this will get more difficult.'

'One day I came back from work and my husband had left a red-hot pan on the stove, then put it on the worktop and the kitchen could have caught fire; that was a signal that he needed 24-hour supervision.'

What family members and friends need to support a person with dementia

To summarise our discussion so far, it is our position that people with dementia can lead lives that are fulfilling and of good quality. Dementia does not have to be a totally distressing and negative condition for a person – they can experience well-being. People with dementia who have a good quality of life, characterised by positive relationships with others and the opportunity to exercise choice and independence and to keep active, may even progress through dementia at a slower rate. Good professional help is necessary for a person with dementia to achieve a good quality of life, but even more vital is the contribution of family members and friends. This places a considerable responsibility on those close to a person with dementia and they need to be properly equipped to take on a caring or supportive role. This section considers the fundamentals needed by family members and friends of a person with dementia.

A POSITIVE ATTITUDE

In the past, our society has had an almost totally negative view of dementia. This stereotype can be traced back to Shakespeare's description of decrepit old age in *As You Like It* as 'second childishness and mere oblivion, sans teeth, sans eyes, sans taste, sans everything'. We have also said that our own attitude towards dementia can often be a negative one.

When faced with the reality of dementia, however, we need to attempt to transcend such thoughts. How we do so will be very individual. For many of us it will be a simple question of continuing concern for someone who has been important to us and whom we love. Others may approach the issue from the perspective of how they would want to be cared for if they themselves developed dementia. However we do it, supporting a person with dementia begins with the assumptions that the person is still a person worthy of our respect and love, and that we can make a positive difference to their quality of life and sense of well-being.

UNDERSTANDING ABOUT DEMENTIA

To successfully support a person with dementia we need to understand their situation. This understanding must be at several levels. First, we need to understand the condition itself. As we will discuss in the next chapter, it is important that a diagnosis is made and that family members and friends know what that diagnosis is, what it is likely to involve for the person and how the condition is likely to progress. We need to know if any medical treatments are available and what effects they might have, and we need to know what the consequences of dementia might be for the person's ongoing physical health as well as their cognitive state.

Second, we need to understand the person themselves, how they are experiencing dementia and how they are feeling about their situation. As discussed earlier, this means we must empathise with the person: we must try to judge their feelings – emotional empathy – and to appreciate how they understand the world – dementia empathy.

SUPPORTING AND CARING SKILLS

Supporting or caring for a person with dementia is a skilled business. We need to know how to interact and communicate with the person, how to help them manage their difficulties while maintaining their independence, and how to respond when their behaviour causes difficulties for us. We also need to adapt our approach as the person's condition progresses. There is no reason to suppose that we will already possess these skills – why should we if we have not known a person with dementia before?

We may draw a parallel here with becoming a parent and having to acquire the skills of childcare. New parents are similarly placed in a situation of having to take on a highly responsible role without prior experience and usually without training. No wonder many new parents buy books on childcare to help them learn the skills they need.

In drawing this parallel, we must of course be very clear about what we are saying. Speaking about people with dementia and children together is fraught with danger because there is the clear risk of belittling or demeaning people with dementia by comparing them with children. Shakespeare's image of 'second childishness' is part of the pervasive negative stereotype that society has regarding dementia. At the same time it is the case that, just as a new parent can learn the skills of childcare, family members and friends of a person with dementia can learn how best to support and care for that person. This is, after all, the purpose of this book.

PEER AND PROFESSIONAL SUPPORT

The final aspect of supporting a person with dementia is to have support oneself in undertaking that role. This support should come both from within the family and one's circle of friends, and also from professional services. We stated earlier that in many cases a particular person becomes main carer for the person with dementia, either willingly or by being more or less thrust into that role. Some of our readers will be in this position, while others will be more concerned with remaining in touch with the person with dementia and supporting the main carer. Whatever your role, a positive attitude towards the person with dementia needs to be accompanied by a positive desire to support one another. Accepting help and support from others is essential both practically and emotionally, whatever your relationship with the person with dementia.

'What you need is someone to talk to face to face, a hug when you are down, or somebody to say, "You are doing fine, you are OK." Encouragement keeps you going.'

'It isn't just the spouse or the family that need support: friends also need support. My friend and I have given each other an enormous amount of support and she has come along to some of the education groups since which have helped her.'

Professional care and support should be available for people with dementia in English-speaking countries at all phases of the journey, but access to professional support and the quality of professional input are ongoing issues worldwide for people with dementia and their families and friends. Some may want the government to provide everything for people with dementia and feel that they should be looked after in hospitals or other residential care settings, paid for out of the public purse, as happened in many countries years ago (one of us began his career working with people with dementia on 'psychogeriatric' wards in a large mental hospital that has long since closed down). While funding arrangements will vary from country to country, there is in all English-speaking countries ongoing debate about how much the government should pay for dementia care and how much the cost should be borne by the person with dementia and their family. We should, however, remember that any discussion about who should provide and pay for dementia care is meaningless to those living in many developing countries where government-funded dementia care, whether residential or in the community, is non-existent and families must fend for themselves.

At its best, professional input at a range of levels can make an important contribution to enhancing the well-being of people with dementia and easing the challenges for families and friends. While specific service provision varies from country to country, we will discuss in later chapters the main types of professional support available at different points in the journey through dementia.

'I needed to have a professional view from someone who can give advice about dementia, tailored to our particular situation. I do not mean someone who would just signpost me to information but somebody with a backpack of knowledge, who could have helped me directly.'

How this book can help

Our aim in this book is to assist family members and friends in acquiring those things they need in order to support a person with dementia and themselves. We will provide basic information about the main types of dementia and their ongoing effects. We will try to help readers appreciate the difficulties of dementia and learn to empathise with the person's feelings and understanding of their world. We will try to enhance readers' skills in interacting with people with dementia in a range of situations and we will outline sources of professional support and how to access it.

What we can't do is give our readers a positive attitude towards people with dementia. That has to come from within.

CHAPTER 2

Someone Close to Me May Have Dementia

Assessment, Diagnosis and Types of Dementia

Identifying dementia

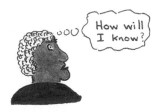

Do you know for sure that someone close to you has dementia? Has the person undergone a formal assessment process and been given a diagnosis by a doctor? If so, it is likely that you will already be familiar with much of the information contained within the early sections of this chapter. You will have gone through the period of uncertainty when the person's cognitive abilities gradually appear to lessen; have undergone the stressful process of assessment and cognitive testing, and eventually have received the news, expected or otherwise, that it is dementia. The difficult journey will have begun, but you will know what is happening and will have some idea what to expect.

You will also be in a minority. Despite improved awareness of dementia, supported by public health campaigns and enhanced specialist assessment and diagnosis, it is still the case that many people with dementia never receive a formal diagnosis, meaning that they and their families are never actually told by a doctor that they have dementia. If you suspect that a person you are close to may have dementia but are unsure what to do next, this chapter may help you understand what is happening to the person and encourage you to seek a proper assessment and diagnosis. As we will see as we go through the chapter, there are significant advantages in doing so.

The first signs of dementia

Many conditions that have far-reaching consequences for a person and those close to them begin with small and apparently trivial signs, and dementia is no exception. Dementia characteristically starts with a person making little mistakes or acting in ways that are a bit unusual for them, but not especially alarming. We all sometimes act in ways that mimic the earliest sign of dementia; consider whether you have ever…

- forgotten the name of a person you know well?

- forgotten an appointment?

- made a cup of tea and then forgotten you have made it?

- in conversation, found it hard to find the right word for a familiar object?

- not been able to identify the day of the week?

- lost your way going to somewhere you've been to before?

- put on the wrong clothes for the weather or inappropriate clothes for the situation?

- found yourself unable to keep track of a conversation you're having?

- forgotten to pay a regular bill?

- put something down and not been able to find it again?

- felt particularly moody or angry and not known why?

- felt that someone else was trying to undermine you or cause you harm, with little evidence that this was the case?

We suspect that many of you will have ruefully admitted that some of these have happened to you at some time. You may well recognise some items on this list as being the first warning signs that all was not well with the person you are now concerned about. The fact that dementia in its earliest phase appears to be little more than day-to-day absent-mindedness or touchiness can make it very hard for families and friends to realise that something is amiss.

> 'It's difficult to say when it started for my mother – at first we thought she was depressed from retiring from work.'

> 'We weren't initially worried as we thought it was his hearing or his sight. He often seemed to be a little bit distant; I'd say something and he wouldn't react, but both his hearing and sight were tested and were fine.'

Eventually however, the person's manner and behaviour become sufficiently unusual and problematic for families and friends to become concerned. The key to recognition of the possibility of dementia may be that there is a noticeable *change* in the person. Perhaps someone whose memory is normally spot on starts to become forgetful or a characteristically cheerful person becomes moody or distracted. The change may alternatively be one of degree – a person may have always been somewhat absent minded or touchy but becomes noticeably more so.

> 'My husband had always been in charge of finances but I went into his office one day and found that he had not been organising his paperwork; things had been opened and not dealt with. I realised he was not taking things in. It was a bit of a shock.'

Stereotypes of old age can hinder recognition of dementia. Our image of an older person may well be of someone who becomes slower on the uptake, forgetful and set in their ways. Nothing could be further from the truth about the majority of older people, but if an older person acts in these ways we may well say 'it's their age' rather than consider the possibility of dementia.

Another factor that may prevent dementia being identified is what we may harshly call 'denial'. None of us wants to contemplate the possibility of a close relative or friend developing dementia, with all the implications that the condition brings with it. If a person we love starts to act in the ways listed earlier, we may make excuses for them, or play down the significance of the way the person's manner is changing. Sometimes this reluctance to face the possibility of dementia can persist long after the signs of the condition are obvious and the person may never receive a formal diagnosis of dementia.

How people with dementia react to the onset of the condition

People in the initial phase of dementia will of course react to their developing condition in a range of ways. Some will interpret their experiences of absent mindedness or moodiness as temporary lapses caused by everyday stresses, or by 'old age creeping on'. Others will be increasingly aware that all is not well but will downplay the issue through 'denial' or hide their growing difficulties from family and friends so as not to alarm them. Others may acknowledge the problem and be willing to seek help.

> 'It was my husband who noticed it and wanted to do something about it. He said, "I'm forgetting things and I think I shouldn't be" – we decided to go to the GP.'

> 'I discovered later that my wife had been to see her best friend and said to her, "I think I've got Alzheimer's." She asked her friend not to say anything to me and she didn't.'

A proportion of people in the first phase of dementia will already begin to lose awareness of their condition and will deny that anything is wrong with them because of a genuine lack of understanding of what is happening to them. This will create further issues for concerned family and friends who may notice changes that the person doesn't see and may try to persuade them to seek help when they don't see the need for it. In such cases diagnosis may be delayed, or families may find themselves resorting to 'white lies' in order to get the person assessed. If you have concerns but the person themselves or others are reluctant to get an assessment, it is important to remember that there are significant benefits to getting a diagnosis. Information leaflets about the process and options for treatment and support may be helpful. Concerns should also be shared with professionals who are clinically responsible for the person, such as the family doctor, because they may have more success in encouraging the person to have an assessment.

Diagnosing dementia

Diagnosis is the process whereby a doctor formally confirms that a person has a particular condition and names that condition. Diagnosis allows treatment to be given, if such exists, and means that the doctor can offer a prognosis – a forecast of how the person's condition may progress and what the future will hold. A diagnosis of a life-changing and terminal condition such as dementia is of course a highly significant event – a watershed in the life of the person and their family and friends; as devastating as a diagnosis of terminal cancer. How that diagnosis is obtained will have a significant bearing on how the person and those close to them face the future.

There is today a systematic process that should be gone through in order to investigate memory or cognitive problems and diagnose dementia. In the first instance the person should consult their family doctor or general practitioner (GP). In some cases the GP will feel confident to assess and diagnose the person themselves, or if available they may refer the person to a memory assessment service (sometimes called a 'memory clinic'). This is a multi-professional service that has the specialised role of assessing, diagnosing and treating such problems. Wherever assessment takes place, the process of investigating for possible dementia is a systematic one:

- A full medical history of the person is taken, including any previous physical or mental health problems.

- A physical examination is carried out, to rule out any treatable causes of the person's symptoms.

- A test of the person's cognitive abilities is carried out.

- The person may be referred for a 'brain scan'.

The centrepiece of assessment is the test of cognitive abilities. This will be administered by the assessor, who will ask the person questions and give them brief tasks to perform. A range of tests are available for the purpose of assessing possible dementia; the best known is called the Mini-Mental State Examination (MMSE), but others may be used.

Cognitive testing is of course a very anxiety-provoking process for both the person and those close to them. Although the tests are brief and the questions simple, it is like taking an examination, the result of which will have far-reaching implications. Testing should be carried out in a sensitive and professional way, with the person given every opportunity to give their best performance – a suggestion that someone has dementia when in fact they do not will not be helpful, given the stigma that dementia can carry.

> 'Mum was angry – she said, "Are they testing to see if I'm stupid?"'

POSSIBLE OUTCOMES OF COGNITIVE ASSESSMENT

In broad terms, there are four possible outcomes:

- It is quite possible that a person's cognitive abilities are found to be 'normal' and there is no indication of dementia.

The person's absent-mindedness may be more apparent than real and the assessment will reassure them that there is no significant problem.

- Investigations may reveal another condition that is causing the person's symptoms. It may be that the person is experiencing *delirium*, a state that can be caused by a number of illnesses in which the person appears to be 'confused' and apparently in the early phase of dementia (it is sometimes called 'acute confusional state'). A wide range of conditions can cause episodes of delirium in older people, in particular infections. Treating the underlying condition should relieve the confusion. Delirium can often be distinguished from dementia by its sudden onset and fluctuations in behaviour. Another condition that can mimic dementia is severe depression. Again, the person may appear to be forgetful and confused, but history taking and sensitive assessment by a professional may reveal that the person is actually very depressed. Treatment of the underlying depression with anti-depressant drugs and other therapies should in time lead to the person's cognitive abilities being restored. Some other rare conditions may also appear like dementia, including some vitamin deficiencies and brain tumours.

- Assessment of the person's cognitive abilities may reveal some deficits, but not enough for a doctor to say for sure that they have dementia. In such cases, the person may be told that they have mild cognitive impairment (MCI). This means exactly what it says: there is evidence of some impairment of the person's cognitive abilities but it cannot be said for sure that the person is in the early phase of dementia. MCI can be caused by a range of factors, including stress and normal ageing, but in some cases it may predict that the person will go on to develop dementia, though it is not possible with current knowledge to identify with certainty who will actually do so.

- The final possible outcome of cognitive assessment is of course that a diagnosis of dementia is made. It may be that the doctor will say simply that the person's condition is 'dementia' or they may feel confident enough to name the actual type of dementia. In whichever case, the journey through dementia has now formally begun for the person and for their family and friends.

Why is diagnosis important and why do many people with dementia not receive a diagnosis?

Before we move on, it is worth considering these questions. If so many people with dementia never receive a diagnosis and apparently get through their lives, why is diagnosis so important? Also, what are the factors that prevent people getting a diagnosis?

The importance of diagnosis for the person and their family is twofold. First, diagnosis creates certainty – the person's experiences and actions can be explained and information can be given. Also, plans can be made for the future – we will talk more about this in the next chapter. Second, diagnosis provides access to professional services and to medical treatment, if available – again, we will discuss currently available treatments later. Professional opinion is virtually unanimous that early assessment and diagnosis of dementia is highly desirable, hence the focus in many countries on building up memory assessment services.

'I think when we were told the diagnosis I felt relief because we'd got a name for what my husband had. I think it was later it became more real. I initially thought now it's got a name, like measles or mumps, I thought, "OK, we can deal with it."'

'I have a good friend who actually divorced her husband because of the problems that his dementia symptoms created. They didn't have a diagnosis for a long time – you can see how the lack of diagnosis actually caused them to divorce.'

But if diagnosis is so important, why do many people never receive a diagnosis? This is a complex question with perhaps as many answers as there are undiagnosed cases of dementia. Some will be people who have lived with dementia for many years and will have developed the condition at a time when diagnosis was afforded less importance. Some families will not have known how to go about getting a diagnosis or professional help and may have muddled along the best they could. Still others may have simply put down the changes in the person to old age. The onset of dementia can often be missed if the person is younger because early signs may be less recognisable and more linked to changes in behaviour and perception than memory loss. Finally, some families may have avoided getting a diagnosis for fear of the stigma that goes with the label of dementia; one person was never diagnosed because her daughter was afraid that diagnosis would have meant her mother would be 'taken away and put in a home'. If readers recognise that they are in any of these categories, we would urge them to contact their GP and arrange for a formal assessment and diagnosis, because even if dementia has progressed there are still benefits to be gained.

Should the person with dementia be told the diagnosis?

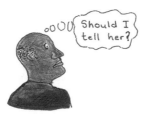

This can be a controversial and sensitive question. Traditionally, it was felt that a person with dementia should not be told about their condition, either because it was thought that they could not take it in or understand its implications, or because they might find the news overwhelming. The result was often a conspiracy of silence in which family and friends avoided the issue when with the person. Some readers may remember that years ago this was often also the case with people who had cancer – it was common for doctors to give the diagnosis of terminal cancer to the person's relatives rather than the person themselves and a similar conspiracy of silence would prevail until the severity of their condition became obvious to the person.

> 'I had suspected what it was and was worried that my wife would spiral down if she was told it was "dementia"; so I asked for them not to use the "D" word.'

> 'I don't think we ever said the word "Alzheimer's" to Mum. I think we said, "Your memory's not good" or something like that. I think I said lots of words about what was happening to her but not that word.'

Today the situation with regard to disclosing a diagnosis of cancer to a person is very different and except in rare circumstances the person will now always receive the diagnosis themselves. There is growing consensus that as a rule the same should be the case for people with dementia. With diagnosis tending to be made at an earlier phase, many people retain awareness and can both take in the news and use it in a positive way, by finding ways of compensating for their difficulties and by contributing to making plans for the future. To be told that they have dementia is of course distressing for the person, and families and friends sometimes want to keep the diagnosis from them to save their feelings, but research indicates that on the whole people with dementia (like people with other life-threatening illnesses) want to know the truth and can cope with the implications of diagnosis.

> 'One day my husband found the book I'd bought on Alzheimer's disease in the filing cabinet. He was reading it in the garden when I came home and he said, "This is it – this is what I've got." We both burst into tears and I put my arms around him and said, "I'll be here for you whatever."'

> 'In one of my husband's diaries he had written: "So it is Alzheimer's; I hope when the end comes, it is not too messy."'

What if a person appears to lack awareness of what is happening to them? Would it be helpful to try to tell them the diagnosis in those circumstances? This is not a straightforward question. Sometimes people with dementia have more awareness than is apparent and can absorb information despite not appearing to do so. At the same time many would say that, if a person has a profound lack of awareness of aspects of their present situation, it is not just futile but cruel to try to orientate them to an unpleasant reality, a point we will return to later in this book.

> 'The diagnosis was very clearly explained to us but when we were with the doctor I looked round and saw that my husband had gone to sleep; he couldn't cope with any long detailed explanations by that time.'

> 'I am not sure my husband can take his diagnosis on intellectually. He tends to see it as being hard for me rather than for himself. He sometimes refers to it now as his "gentle lunacy."'

After the diagnosis

Research has highlighted what people newly diagnosed with dementia, and their family and friends, need at that point in the journey. An initial key need is for information, about dementia as a concept, about the specific disease that the person has, and about the skills and qualities that families and friends require in order to help the person. Second, there is the need for access to support, both practical and emotional, for the person and for those close to them. Third, there is the need to plan for the future, because the time will inevitably come when the person will not be able to care for themselves and will need help and care from others. Finally, if possible, medical treatment needs to be prescribed that may in some cases slow the progression of the condition.

Unfortunately, it is not always the case that these needs are met effectively by professional services. Many people with dementia and their families report being more or less abandoned by professionals once the diagnosis has been made, with little advice or support other than a general 'contact your GP if you have any problems'. People in the early phase of dementia, and their families and friends, are often left to fend for themselves, a state of affairs that is increasingly being regarded as unacceptable in political and professional circles.

> 'I was given a leaflet but had really nobody to talk to. We were just sort of shown out into the street.'

As we will see in Chapter 3, some initiatives are being developed to provide more help for families during what we call 'the gap years' and knowing how to access such help is important. But in the rest of this chapter and the next chapter of this book, we will attempt to provide some of the basic information and advice that is needed once the diagnosis of dementia has been confirmed.

The main types of dementia

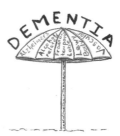

As we suggested earlier, a principal need of people with dementia and their families and friends following diagnosis is information about their condition. In the case of dementia, this means both information about the broad syndrome of dementia (discussed in the last chapter) and information about the specific type of dementia that the person has, provided that a particular type has been identified. There are over a hundred types of dementia, the majority extremely rare, and we won't try to list every one in this book. In this section and the next we will, however, say something about the most common types of dementia. We will start with those that generally lead to late-onset dementia (when signs and symptoms first appear after the age of 65).

ALZHEIMER'S DISEASE

This is the most common type of dementia and is sometimes equated with dementia – in several countries the leading dementia charities feature Alzheimer's disease in their titles (the Alzheimer's Society in the UK, the Alzheimer's Association in the USA and Alzheimer's Australia). Alzheimer's disease has the features most often associated with dementia. It usually begins with memory problems, the person particularly having difficulty remembering newly learnt information. Memory deficits gradually worsen and other signs of dementia start to appear, such as problems with language, orientation, attention and carrying out daily tasks (executive function). The development of difficulties happens slowly, over a period of months or years, the person eventually slipping from 'early' through 'moderate' to 'advanced' dementia, becoming more and more dependent on others.

Alzheimer's disease is a neurodegenerative disorder, meaning that it is caused by the degeneration and death of cells in the brain (neurons), particularly in the cortex – the grey matter that makes up the surface of the brain. This causes the brain of an affected person to *atrophy*: it shrinks, losing weight and volume as cells gradually die. The biochemical processes that lead to the degeneration of brain cells are highly complex and not well understood and are beyond the scope of this book. However, two things happen to affected brain cells that together are diagnostic features of Alzheimer's disease. First, large numbers of *plaques* develop within diseased cells. These are deposits of a protein called 'beta-amyloid' and can be seen under a powerful microscope. Second, *neurofibrillary tangles* are found within the same cells. These are deposits of another substance called 'tau protein', which under the microscope appear like tightly tangled threads. Medical experts disagree with each other about the relative influence of beta-amyloid and tau in causing the death of brain cells. Recent research has indicated that the process of neurodegeneration can begin many years before the person starts to show the signs of Alzheimer's disease.

Alzheimer's disease is the most common type of dementia in people with Down's syndrome (see Chapter 1). Typically the age of onset of the condition is earlier than in the population as a whole. Around 2 per cent of people with Down's syndrome will show the signs and symptoms of dementia in their 30s, rising to over 50 per cent of those in their 60s.

Treatment and progression of Alzheimer's disease

As with other types of dementia, there is currently no treatment for Alzheimer's disease that will lead to a cure or will stop the continual process of brain cell degeneration and death. There are, however, some drugs that may delay the progression of Alzheimer's disease for a time, and which can be prescribed following diagnosis by a doctor or a memory assessment service. This group of drugs is called 'acetylcholinesterase inhibitors' (ACEIs – sometimes simply called 'anti-dementia drugs'). These drugs can compensate for the loss of a brain chemical called 'acetylcholine', which plays a role in memory and other cognitive functions. Three drugs are available within this group: donepezil (marketed in the UK as Aricept), rivastigmine (Exelon) and galantamine (Reminyl). All work in slightly different ways and have slightly different side effects, and one drug may suit a person better than another. Also, some people who take the drugs find that they do not gain much benefit from them. While the ACEI drugs may be limited in what they offer, many people with dementia and their families appreciate the benefits that they can bring.

Another drug, called memantine (Ebixa), is also available. This works in a different way from the ACEI drugs and is recommended for relief of symptoms in people with moderate to advanced dementia. Again, its benefits are modest, but evidence suggests that it may help make some people feel less agitated and make their behaviour less difficult for others.

Research is being carried out worldwide to try to find better treatments for dementia, but many in the field complain that less money is put into dementia research than into other life-limiting conditions such as cancer. Current opinion is that there is unlikely to be a 'cure' for Alzheimer's disease in the near future, or anything that will prevent Alzheimer's disease from taking hold. However, some researchers feel that that the future is more optimistic and predict new curative and preventative treatments being available in the next ten years. What is clear is that we are learning more about dementia and there is hope that further research will lead to new solutions.

The long-term prognosis of Alzheimer's disease, as with other illnesses that lead to dementia, is for increasing difficulties leading eventually to death. How long a person will live with the condition will be very variable and, because a large number of people will not show symptoms until very late in life, many will die from other age-related illnesses before they reach the phase of advanced dementia. It is quite possible, however, for a person to live for a number of years with the condition.

VASCULAR DEMENTIA

As the name suggests, vascular dementia is caused by cerebral-vascular disease – that is, disease of blood and its circulation around the brain. Vascular dementia is itself a syndrome and there are several specific diseases that are included within the term. In all cases, however, vascular dementia is caused by disease or damage to the blood vessels that supply brain cells, leading to loss of blood supply and consequent damage and death of brain tissue. The three most common forms of vascular dementia are:

- Multi-infarct dementia: in this condition, a person experiences a series of 'mini-strokes' or transient ischaemic attacks (TIAs). Each time the person experiences a TIA, another small area of brain tissue is damaged, causing loss of cognitive function in that area. Eventually, if TIAs happen frequently enough, the grey matter of the brain becomes sufficiently damaged for the signs and symptoms of dementia to become apparent.

- Single-infarct dementia: in rare cases, a person who has had just one large stroke may afterwards display all the signs and symptoms of dementia, if the stroke occurred in a particularly important area of the brain.

- Small vessel disease-related dementia: also called 'sub-cortical vascular dementia' or 'Binswanger's disease', this condition results from damage to blood vessels deep inside the brain.

VASCULAR DEMENTIA AND ALZHEIMER'S DISEASE COMPARED

The onset and progression of vascular dementia may vary from those of Alzheimer's disease. Sometimes its onset is relatively sudden, reflecting the fact that a person has had a stroke or a TIA. Sometimes the condition progresses in a 'step-wise' pattern, in which the person may experience an abrupt onset of symptoms followed by a relatively long period of stability. The person then experiences another small stroke that leads to another increase in symptoms, and that pattern continues over a period of months or years until the difficulties become profound. The nature of the person's difficulties may be very individual; unlike Alzheimer's disease in which there is often a general increase in difficulties in all areas of a person's cognitive life, with vascular dementia some abilities may be profoundly affected at an early phase while others are preserved, reflecting the specific areas of the brain that have been damaged by each stroke.

At the same time, there is a complex relationship between vascular dementia and Alzheimer's disease. Many people turn out to have elements of both conditions – they will be experiencing both the degeneration of brain cells that is characteristic of Alzheimer's disease and the damage to blood vessels in the brain that causes vascular dementia. Without a brain scan it can often be difficult for doctors to determine which condition a person has – or the relative balance of Alzheimer's disease and vascular dementia. Current evidence suggests that, while Alzheimer's disease is the most common single form of dementia, around 50 per cent of people with dementia will have some cerebral-vascular disease, either vascular dementia or 'mixed dementia', including elements of both Alzheimer's disease and vascular dementia.

Treatment and progression of vascular dementia

There is no way with our current state of knowledge that the brain damage that characterises vascular dementia can be reversed. However, it is possible that vascular dementia may be prevented, or its progression slowed down or halted if factors that lead to the underlying vascular disease are addressed. The risk of vascular disease can be significantly reduced by maintaining a healthy body weight, eating a diet that minimises saturated fats and includes lots of fruit, vegetables and fish, drinking alcohol within safe limits, not smoking and taking regular exercise. Getting treatment for vascular-related conditions such as hypertension (high blood pressure) or diabetes will also reduce risk. If the signs and symptoms of vascular dementia do appear, adopting a healthy lifestyle and treating underlying vascular disease can slow or even stop the progression of the condition – it is possible for people to have a number of mini-strokes (TIAs) without vascular dementia developing.

Current opinion is that the ACEI drugs developed to treat Alzheimer's disease are not effective for people with vascular dementia, though they may be prescribed for mixed dementia. If underlying vascular factors are not brought under control, vascular dementia may progress until the person experiences advanced dementia and will lead to their death. As with Alzheimer's disease, this process may take some years.

DEMENTIA WITH LEWY BODIES

This is the third main type of late-onset dementia, though it is probably less common than Alzheimer's disease or vascular dementia. Like Alzheimer's disease, it involves degeneration and death of brain cells, leading to a generally gradual, progressive increase in difficulties, though memory is sometimes less affected in the early phase. A person with dementia with Lewy bodies may also have periods of drowsiness or faintness and may be prone to falls. They may experience visual hallucinations, false perceptions when they believe they can see things that are not really there. Finally, the person may display signs of Parkinsonism, including stiffness of joints and limbs and tremor in limbs that they cannot control. If brain cells of a person with dementia with Lewy bodies are examined under a microscope, Lewy bodies are seen within them. These are spherical protein deposits (also found in Parkinson's disease) that, through a process that is not well understood, lead to death of the cell.

Treatment and progression of dementia with Lewy bodies

There is at present no known way of preventing dementia with Lewy bodies and no known cure. It is possible that ACEI drugs may be useful in slowing the progression of dementia with Lewy bodies, but at present the evidence for this is not strong. Dementia with Lewy bodies will inevitably lead to progressive difficulties and eventual death.

It is important, however, to accurately diagnose dementia with Lewy bodies because some sedating drugs that are sometimes used to attempt to reduce aggressive or agitated behaviour in people with dementia may have particularly severe side effects if given to a person with this condition (see Chapter 5).

Young-onset dementia

The main late-onset dementias – Alzheimer's disease, vascular dementia and dementia with Lewy bodies – can also occur in people under the age of 65. Many other diseases can cause dementia in younger people (while also occasionally appearing for the first time when a person is over 65). Almost all are progressive and incurable and, however the disease begins, the person will eventually experience the profound difficulties of advanced dementia. In the early phase, though, different types may have their own particular features. Some will have related physical problems, particularly affecting a person's ability to use their muscles.

We saw in the last chapter that around 17,000 people in the UK and 200,000 in the USA have a diagnosis of young-onset dementia, defined as dementia that manifests itself before the age of 65. These figures are likely to be substantial under-estimates – some research suggests that there may actually be around three times that number, with many cases undiagnosed. If recognising late-onset dementia is difficult in the early phase, identifying dementia in younger people is often considerably harder, for two main reasons. First, because of its rarity, dementia is not expected to occur in younger people and therefore, if a person is appearing to think or act in unusual ways, they or their families and friends are likely to attribute their signs and symptoms to other factors, such as stress or other mental or physical disorders. Second, the early signs of several types of young-onset dementia are often not the same as those of late-onset dementias, leading again to possible misidentification. Another factor that suggests there are more under 65s with dementia than are known to have the condition is the growing evidence from neuro-imaging studies that the underlying brain disease that causes late-onset dementia may begin some years before the person starts to show any signs and symptoms, implying that there may be many under 65s who are already harbouring dementia without knowing it.

> 'I think there are huge difficulties for younger people with getting a diagnosis. They are often diagnosed with depression, and you can go with the tablets and a year or more goes by and nothing happens.'

The following are some of the more prevalent young-onset conditions, though all are extremely uncommon.

YOUNG-ONSET ALZHEIMER'S DISEASE

Alzheimer's disease is the most common young-onset dementia, accounting for around one-third of all cases of dementia in those under the age of 65. Indeed, Dr Alois Alzheimer's first published case description in 1907 of the disease that bears his name was of a woman in her early 50s. Alzheimer's disease has the same features in younger people as in those who are in later life and the condition progresses in the same way. ACEI drugs may help younger people for a time. There appears to be a sub-type of Alzheimer's disease that affects younger people that has a strongly genetic element to it, with several members of the same family affected by the condition.

FRONTO-TEMPORAL DEMENTIA

This term covers a number of conditions, including Pick's disease, frontal lobe degeneration and dementia associated with muscular dystrophy. All are degenerative conditions that lead to death of brain cells, though the underlying causes are not well understood. Each begins in the frontal and temporal lobes of the cortex – the area of grey matter at the front and on each side of the brain. These areas are predominantly concerned with governing our social abilities, executive function, behaviour and language skills, and it is these aspects that are initially affected rather than memory. The first signs of the condition are therefore often moodiness or inexplicable lapses in social etiquette – for example, a normally very polite lady would suddenly say to one of us as part of a routine conversation, 'Your breath stinks.' As the condition progresses, the person's manner may change; they may become either much more subdued or more outgoing than before. Social lapses may become more prominent, the person perhaps becoming quite aggressive or rude, or sometimes sexually disinhibited. Such behaviour is clearly very difficult for families and friends to understand and cope with, but it is important when this happens that others realise that the person 'can't help it' – it is purely an effect of the disease process.

HUNTINGTON'S DISEASE

This is a disease that affects both the areas of the brain that govern thinking and mental life and also parts of the brain that regulate the motor nerves that control the action of muscles. This means that the person has progressive difficulties in movement and the use of muscles as well as developing dementia. Huntington's disease is caused by a single dominant gene, which means that a child of a person with the condition has a 50 per cent chance of developing the illness themselves. The first signs of the condition usually appear when the person is in their 30s. The person will develop 'tics' or involuntary muscular movements, and their manner may start to change; they may become moody and sometimes uncontrollably aggressive. Cognitive difficulties include issues with short-term memory and concentration.

As the disease progresses, the person experiences increasing problems with involuntary movements and also weight loss. Cognitive difficulties also increase and the person can be particularly prone to mood swings, depression and stubbornness. As time goes on, dementia becomes more advanced. People can live with Huntington's disease for 10 to 20 years and in some countries there are a few specialist residential units to care for people with the condition, given the profound physical as well as mental symptoms that come with it.

ALCOHOL-RELATED DEMENTIA

Alcohol can lead to dementia in more than one way. It is a toxin that can damage brain cells and excessive consumption over many years can sometimes cause enough damage to lead to dementia (this condition is called 'alcoholic dementia'). More commonly, people who misuse alcohol risk developing *Korsakoff's syndrome*, which is a dementia-like condition that results from a deficiency in vitamin B12, a state that heavy drinkers can be prone to find themselves in. If the underlying vitamin deficiency is identified and treated at an early stage, the symptoms of confusion and disorientation can be relieved, but unfortunately the lifestyles of those who excessively misuse alcohol often prevent them from accessing such medical attention and their difficulties can become permanent.

All in all, moderating our alcohol consumption is an important step in reducing our risk of developing dementia. Although few of us drink heavily or recklessly enough to develop alcohol-related dementia, as we have seen, drinking above safe limits increases the risk for all of us of vascular disease, which in turn is a strong factor in the development of both vascular dementia and Alzheimer's disease.

CREUTZFELDT-JACOB DISEASE

Creutzfeldt-Jacob disease (CJD) is a very rare condition that leads to a rapidly progressive dementia, with profound cognitive and physical difficulties and death usually within two years of onset of symptoms. It is known to be caused by the presence in brain tissue of mutated *prions*. Prions are proteins that are integral parts of cells, but in their mutated form they can cause cell death. People with CJD have either experienced mutation of prions within their own brains, or have been infected by mutated prions from another source. In recent years a new form of CJD has been identified, especially in the UK, known as 'variant CJD'. This appears to have been caused by people eating meat from cattle infected by bovine spongiform encephalopathy (BSE), a disease of cattle that is also caused by mutated prions. BSE was prevalent in the UK in the late 1980s and early 1990s and quantities of infected meat entered the food chain, ending up particularly in processed foods such as beefburgers. Consequently, those who have developed variant CJD have tended to be quite young. Stringent regulations have now eliminated BSE from cattle destined for human consumption and the incidence of new cases of variant CJD seems to be slowing down, but it is not known how many people have been infected by mutated prions from cattle with BSE and it is still possible that there may be an epidemic of variant CJD in the UK in years to come.

Neurological diseases that may include dementia among their symptoms

A number of conditions that are usually grouped within the medical speciality of neurology may in their late phases lead to dementia-like symptoms as well as to increasing physical disability. These include Parkinson's disease, multiple sclerosis and muscular dystrophy, among others. Dementia may also occur in the late phase of AIDS, though, in Western countries at least, new drug treatments have improved the life expectancy of those with HIV infection and reduced the extent of AIDS- or HIV-related dementia.

CHAPTER 3

Beginning the Journey

The Early Phase of Dementia

The characteristics of early dementia

As we discussed in the previous chapter, it can be difficult to identify and diagnose dementia precisely in the early or 'mild' phase, because its deficits can be attributed to 'normal' ageing. Also, each person will be different, depending on the type of dementia they have and their individual coping strategies. However, a person with early dementia is likely to have some characteristic cognitive issues of the type discussed at the beginning of Chapter 2.

These difficulties will cause real problems with managing daily life. Problems experienced with planning, organising and carrying out complex tasks will compromise a person's ability to work or carry out usual activities, such as hobbies or voluntary work. The increasing forgetfulness will also affect the person's daily life if they forget appointments or neglect important obligations such as paying bills. Family members and friends may well notice the person's mood and behaviour in social situations changing, with the person becoming perhaps distant and withdrawn, finding it harder to contribute to conversation or activities.

'We had always been fairly equal in our relationship but I began to notice changes in my husband's behaviour; like not sharing responsibilities in the house, housework, cooking.'

'My wife would go into herself, and would get quite upset and miserable. She didn't want to go out, she cried quite a bit and she didn't look after herself quite so well. She had always been immaculate, very smart, but she wasn't doing her hair quite right, wasn't doing her make-up quite so well. She also pulled out of doing things; she wasn't meeting up with people or inviting people around.'

Despite this, the person will usually still be able to look after themselves, being able to keep clean, nourished and use the toilet independently. Participation in social interaction and activities remains important and continuing to live independently, if that is what the person was doing before, should still be possible. Even activities such as driving are not impossible in the early phase of dementia. Also, the person will often retain awareness of their situation and still be able to contribute to family discussions and decisions about their future living and care arrangements. However, the person is likely to need the assistance and support of family and friends in order to maintain aspects of their usual lifestyle for as long as possible. In the rest of this chapter, we will examine how family members and friends can help a person in the early phase of dementia and how they can maintain their accustomed relationships with the person.

Dementia empathy and early dementia

Many of us have some longstanding cognitive 'difficulties' that mirror aspects of early dementia:

- People A have chronically poor memories. They regard themselves and are regarded by others as 'absent minded' and frequently forget appointments or fail to recognise people they have met before.

- People B have a very poor sense of direction. They find it hard to understand maps and often lose their way when driving to unfamiliar places.

- People C find it hard to take in complex information. They struggle to understand bureaucratic processes and often fill in official forms wrongly.

- People D find it hard to make difficult decisions. They feel overwhelmed with the various conflicting facts and opinions that they are bombarded with on the matter in question and 'can't see the wood for the trees'.

- People E find interacting with their physical environment hard. They struggle to understand how things relate to each other or fit together. If such a person tries to carry out such things as Do-it-Yourself (DIY) activities or car repairs, they often go horribly wrong.

- People F find reading and writing hard and may have been diagnosed with dyslexia.

Few of us understand the world around us perfectly, or feel completely confident in responding appropriately to all the demands the world places on us. As we discussed in Chapter 2, none of these things are themselves diagnostic of dementia, they simply reflect normal human variability. We would only become concerned and suspect dementia if we perceived a significant unexplained change in our cognitive abilities – a noticeable decline in ability from whatever level we were accustomed to.

We can, however, draw on our own experiences when considering how we might empathise with and support a person in the early phase of dementia. How do we feel about our own cognitive shortcomings? Perhaps we laugh them off or even exaggerate them for effect. On the other hand, we may be more or less distressed and angry with ourselves and regard our difficulties as signs of weakness. Perhaps we will deny that there are things that we aren't good at and put huge efforts into trying to do those things, every failure making us more determined to try again. People with early dementia may react to their own growing difficulties in any of these ways.

Also, how do we compensate for those cognitive difficulties we ourselves experience? Some of us have found strategies for helping us do things we find hard. The forgetful person has learnt to write down reminders, set alarms and keep lists of things they have to do. When meeting a person in the street whom they don't immediately recognise, they may use basic social skills to interact with the person while pretending that they know who they are talking to. The person with a poor sense of direction writes themselves clear instructions for their journey before setting out – or gratefully purchases the latest satnav! The dyslexic person may have acquired aids to reading and writing such as large-print books and word processors to avoid having to handwrite.

In other cases we seek the advice or assistance of others. The person faced with a complex bureaucratic form may go through it with a friend who has completed the same form previously. The person faced with a complicated decision may talk it through with family, or consult a counsellor. The clumsy person will enlist the help of someone more competent to assist with carrying out a DIY task. Ultimately, of course, we may decide that the thing we are struggling with is too hard for us and we decide to either not bother with it or ask someone else to do it for us, either as a favour or in a paid capacity (for example, one of us long ago gave up his unequal struggle with home and car maintenance and now pays through the nose for those things to be done for him!).

Again, people with early dementia will employ any or all of these strategies when managing their own difficulties. In some cases it is possible for a person to continue to do things themselves by modifying their way of doing them, sometimes with the assistance of technology. In other cases a person may still be able to contribute towards getting things done, but will need the help of others in order to successfully fulfil the task.

> 'Dad made a list for getting dressed, what to put on first and what next and Mum followed that for a long time.'

Equally it may be that it is best for a person to give up certain activities and allow others to take them over. These can be difficult decisions, especially if the person is giving up something they value, or lacks awareness that they are not able to perform as they used to.

For family members and friends the aim is to offer just enough help to enable the person with dementia to live their life successfully and safely without taking away the person's independence unnecessarily. Achieving this balance can clearly be hard. How do we know that a person is unable to do something unless they try to do it? But what if they attempt an activity, find they are unable to do it and come to harm as a result? Also, the person's ability to be independent will depend on the nature of the activity – they may be able to carry out some activities without any problem but may struggle with others. Equally, of course, the person's abilities will change over time. Family members and friends need to know the person very well in order to judge when to give help or when to allow the person to continue to do things for themselves – and sometimes have to cross their fingers and hope for the best.

Awareness and capacity in early dementia

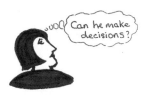

We have discussed in Chapter 1 the idea of awareness in dementia and we have suggested that often people in the early phase of dementia retain considerable awareness both of the world around them and of their own difficulties. This is an appropriate time to introduce a related concept, that of *capacity* (also known in some countries as 'mental capacity' or 'legal capacity'). This is a legal term that governs both what people with dementia can do for themselves in a legal sense and what others, particularly family members and friends, can legally do for them or on their behalf. Capacity is also a useful concept in assisting us with dementia empathy in the early phase of dementia because it is closely linked with the idea of awareness and can help us decide what level of support a person may need at a given time with specific activities.

Most English-speaking countries have passed legislation related to capacity, though the precise nature of that legislation (and some of the legal terminology used) will vary from country to country. Sources of information about legislation in a range of countries can be found in the list of relevant organisations in the 'Resources for Family and Friends' section at the end of this book.

THE CONCEPT OF CAPACITY

'Capacity' is related to the ability to perceive and understand the world accurately and to make decisions and respond to events and circumstances in a considered and appropriate way. In short, people who have capacity 'know what they are doing' – however they are behaving they are doing so with understanding of the situation and having consciously decided to act in that way. It may be that in some cases others would not act in that way or would not have made that decision and may find a person's behaviour strange, but if the person knows what they are doing… they have capacity.

Some people will lack capacity (this is sometimes called 'incapacity'). It is not just people with dementia who may lack capacity: members of other groups including people with learning disabilities, people with acquired brain injury and some people with mental and physical health problems may also lack capacity in the legal sense. Capacity is not a global concept but specific to situations and times, so a person may lack capacity related to some aspects of their life but not to others, or may lack capacity at a certain time (for example, when acutely mentally ill) and may regain capacity in the future. Each country will have a specific legal test for determining if a person should be regarded as lacking capacity.

The capacity of people with dementia to make decisions will be compromised because dementia damages cognitive abilities. However, it must not be assumed that all people with dementia lack capacity in the legal sense – many people with early dementia will pass the legal tests where they are living at least some of the time. This has important implications for family members and friends of a person with dementia not only for ensuring that they keep within the law but also because it enshrines a fundamental ethical stance. We should presume that a person retains capacity to make their own decisions unless it is clear that they cannot. We should do what we can to help the person make their own decisions, or contribute to those decisions, if it is possible for them to do so. Even if their decision is not one we would prefer them to make, we must not assume that it results from a lack of capacity. Finally, if it is decided that the person does lack capacity and that others should make decisions for them, then those decisions must be made in the person's best interests, maintaining as much independence for the person as possible.

We can see how the concepts of mental capacity and awareness are linked – though again we should not regard them as one and the same. However, we can certainly say that the more a person appears to retain awareness of their world and their condition the more likely they are to retain the capacity to make decisions – even if family members and friends don't always agree with the decisions they make.

Planning for the future

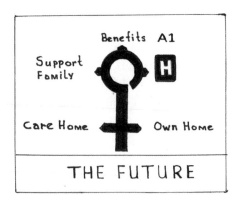

'If I'd known more about what to expect, my husband and I could have had a "whale of a time" whilst it was possible. We would have been able to plan ahead.'

Once dementia has been diagnosed, it is important that the person, their family and friends make plans for the future. Dementia will inevitably progress and key decisions will have to be made regarding such matters as how the person's financial affairs will be managed, where the person will live as their ability to be independent declines and what kind of medical treatment and care they should receive as they approach the end of life. As dementia progresses, they will lose the capacity to make those decisions for themselves. If that is the case and they have not expressed their views in advance, then family members and/or professionals will have to decide for them, in their best interests. However, the decision-making process can be made much easier if discussions have taken place before the person loses capacity, so that they can express their views as to how they would like the rest of their life to proceed.

> 'Don't wait for the future to happen because when it happens you're upset, you're distraught, you don't want to be making the big decisions then.'

> 'We never had a chance to talk about this because earlier on. I didn't realise it was a terminal illness, and I left it too late.'

Such discussions with family members and friends may be informal and unstructured. Family members often say to professionals, 'We talked about it and this is what he would have wanted.' Professionals should take note of such remembered conversations when making decisions, but it is better if the person sets out their views formally in a way that is normally legally binding. In most English-speaking countries, there are two legal mechanisms for a person with dementia to have their wishes taken into account: *advanced decisions* and *power of attorney*.

ADVANCED DECISIONS

An advanced decision (sometimes known as an 'advanced directive' or 'living will') is a legally drawn-up statement of the person's wishes regarding certain future medical treatments or aspects of health care, should they lack capacity to make decisions at the time they need those treatments. The person may decide that they do not want to have treatments such as specific drugs or surgical treatments that would prolong their life, or cardio-pulmonary resuscitation if they have a cardiac arrest. Equally, the person may give permission for certain care strategies to be used, such as the use of assistive technology or admission to residential care. So long as they are valid and applicable, advanced decisions are generally legally binding on professionals. A person can only draw up an advanced decision for themselves and must have mental capacity when doing so, but as stated earlier this may well include many people with early dementia.

Advanced decisions must be drawn up with care so that doctors and nurses in the future have clear guidelines to follow. An advanced decision might say, 'I do not want any form of surgery if I am near the end of my life.' However, it is possible that the person may be in extreme pain and that surgery would make their last months easier for them. It is recommended that people compiling advanced decisions look carefully at the legal principles that prevail where they live, and seek medical and legal advice.

POWER OF ATTORNEY

This principle states that a person can legally appoint another to look after their financial affairs, and/or make other decisions on their behalf once they lack capacity to do so. These decisions may embrace consent to medical treatment, deciding where the person should live and so on. Again, each country will have specific legislation but generally the person must have mental capacity in order to make a power of attorney so it should again ideally be done before the person develops dementia. However, as with advanced decisions, it is still legally possible for someone with early dementia to nominate a family member or friend to take on power of attorney – so long as the person with dementia still has mental capacity.

Taking out power of attorney related to financial matters has obvious advantages in that the attorney can use the person's money to manage their financial affairs and help pay for support and care when the person themselves is unable to do so. It can also help people with dementia living alone avoid being exploited by unscrupulous tradesmen who may try to sell them things or services that they do not need and which would become a financial burden to them.

The legal processes discussed earlier are involved and complex, and so they should be – the potential for a power of attorney to be abused or an advanced decision to be misinterpreted are considerable. But the alternative is that family members, friends and professionals are left guessing what the person would have wanted – and may well guess wrong.

ASSISTED SUICIDE

Although this is an end of life issue and we will discuss end of life care in Chapter 8, we will consider this emotive subject here because it is in the phase of early dementia that a person may particularly wish to consider this option. Few of us relish the prospect of dementia and the potential years of decline, loss of abilities and dignity, and the burden on family members and friends that the condition may bring. One often hears people saying that if they were in that situation they wouldn't want to go on. Some might wish to include directions regarding assisted suicide in an advanced decision.

> 'If Grandma could choose whether to wake up tomorrow or not I think she'd say she's had a good run at things and she wouldn't want to go into a care home.'

Assisted suicide is of course illegal in the UK and in most English-speaking countries. Should the law be changed to allow people with dementia the possibility of assisted suicide? In the UK the author Terry Pratchett, who has a rare form of dementia, has been campaigning for such a change in the law. We may feel that in a modern, liberal society everyone should have the right to end their lives at a time of their choosing, particularly if they have dementia, and the early phase of dementia is the best time to take that decision.

There are, however, two problems with allowing assisted suicide for people with dementia. The first relates to awareness, capacity and consent. If assisted suicide were to be allowed, when should the act be carried out – while a person still has awareness and capacity, or after awareness has gone? If the person still has awareness, they may not want to die. Also, how can one be sure that at the point of deciding to die the person still retained awareness and capacity? On the other hand, if the act of ending the person's life is delayed until the person has lost awareness, then they become unable to change their mind. What if they appear to be quite content with their life – should family members still carry out the person's previously stated wish?

The second problem is perhaps more significant than the first. It relates to the very real fear that people with dementia may covertly or overtly feel pressurised into saying that they will end their lives. We are bombarded by the media with stories about the possible problems that rising numbers of people with dementia will cause society in the future and the financial strain this may cause. Older people may be anxious to be able to leave money to their families rather than see it swallowed up by the costs of caring for them.

Some would take the view that such a state of affairs would be intolerable. Leading charities such as the Alzheimer's Society in the UK and the Alzheimer's Association in the USA hold that wealthy, civilised societies should be prioritising care and support for needy members of those societies, such as people with dementia, not encouraging them to end their lives for the benefit of others. We will leave the last word on this subject to the former UK Prime Minister, Gordon Brown, who in a debate in Parliament on the topic in 2008 said:

> I believe that it's necessary to ensure that there is never a case in the country where a sick or elderly person feels under pressure to agree to an assisted death or somehow feels it's the expected thing to do. (*The Independent* 2008)

Maintaining relationships and keeping active in the phase of early dementia

During the phase of early dementia it should be possible for a person to continue with the relationships and friendships that they already have and to continue to carry out many of their accustomed leisure activities, especially if they retain a level of awareness. At the same time, family members and friends will need to adapt to the person's developing difficulties if this is to happen. It is important for the continued well-being of a person with early dementia that family members and friends understand and apply three broad principles:

1. Inclusion.

2. Assistance.

3. Acceptance.

It is important that efforts are made to *include* the person in social and leisure activities. The person may well need to be *assisted* to carry out their accustomed activities, or to partake in social occasions. Finally, family members and friends may need to display a measure of *acceptance* if the person's difficulties lead to their experiencing problems in social situations, or in carrying out activities. We will consider these principles in more detail.

INCLUSION

A person with dementia cannot maintain social relationships or carry out activities unless they are actively included by family members and friends. This does not always happen. Research has shown that people with dementia can often become 'socially excluded', leading to isolation, impoverished lives and perhaps swifter progression of their condition. Friends and even family members may avoid social contact with the person, through awkwardness, lack of understanding of how to interact with the person or concern regarding the contrast between how the person is now compared with how they used to be. Stigma and prejudice within society can reinforce these socially excluding attitudes.

Inclusion has both a practical and a social component, but these are closely interlinked. The simple fact is that for a person with dementia to *feel* socially included they have to *be* socially included – family members and friends must make the effort to include the person in what they are doing and help the person to continue with their accustomed activities. The person should continue to receive invitations to social events, and family and friends must accept invitations from the person. The person should be allowed to still do activities or to be part of clubs and societies. Most people with early dementia will have retired from full-time employment but they may still carry out voluntary work and may be able to continue with that work.

> 'My husband's diagnosis was devastating for our future plans but I was keen to keep life as normal as possible. I have always needed to go out and made sure we still did this as much as possible.'

> 'My dad took my mum out a lot, he never hid her. Even towards the end when she was in a wheelchair he would take her out. He'd take her to a country pub sometimes. It was important to him.'

The role of friends is crucial in ensuring that a person with early dementia continues to feel included. As stated earlier, friends often drift away from the person, or leave the responsibility of supporting the person to family members. We can sometimes be 'easy come, easy go' when it comes to friendships and social relationships. However, as the saying goes, 'a friend in need is a friend indeed', and few are needier than people with dementia.

> 'As time has gone on it's made a lot of difference to social relations. We have a lot of friends who don't find it easy especially as my husband's behaviour has become more difficult. Other friends have become closer and offer to sit with my husband and that's really important. Some friends and neighbours have drifted away.'

It is also the case that people with dementia may well need practical help in remaining socially included. This can be as simple as having someone collect them and take them home again if they are no longer able to drive. Again, family members and friends may need to make some effort to involve the person in family and social life.

ASSISTANCE

As well as practical assistance with getting to and from social events and activities, people with early dementia may also need assistance from others with actually participating in those events and activities, because of the cognitive difficulties they are experiencing. If this is the case, family members and friends need to display the principles of dementia empathy discussed in Chapter 1. If a person with dementia is experiencing difficulty with participating or socialising, one should endeavour to understand the nature of the person's problems and try and find ways of compensating. As we pointed out in Chapter 1, difficulties may arise with the person's understanding of the world around them, or with their ability to respond appropriately to events in their world.

Difficulties in understanding the world in the early phase of dementia

For many people, a feature of early dementia is likely to be memory loss, a person having particular difficulty remembering new information but also sometimes forgetting things that they would previously have remembered as a matter of routine, such as paying a bill on time or taking their key with them when going out. Sometimes the person might forget where they are when away from their home and not be able to find their way home. Family members and friends can assist them by providing memory aids. These might include drawing up lists of things the person must remember to do, phoning or texting them with reminders of appointments or drawing clear directions to help the person get about. It should be anticipated that the person might not remember things said to them and we should be prepared to repeat ourselves, or write down important messages. Mobile phones, provided the person understands how to use them, can be valuable aids that families and friends can use to send the person reminders and also as a source of help in emergencies.

There are an increasing number of what are referred to as 'assistive technology devices' that can help support someone's independence (see later).

Difficulties with responding to the world in the early phase of dementia

A person's memory difficulties will clearly affect their ability to respond to events in their world. It may be as simple as the person not remembering the name of someone who is talking to them, or forgetting an appointment. They may forget to take important medicines. Again, tactful reminders are helpful and will be appreciated by the person.

The person may begin to experience difficulties with maintaining attention and carrying out complex tasks (executive function). This may lead to their struggling to keep up with others in conversations or when taking part in some activities or hobbies. Family members and friends may assist by recognising where the person has problems, offering guidance and, if possible, making the activity simpler. It is easy to overestimate the cognitive abilities of a person with early dementia because the person is likely to retain superficial social skills – for example, they may put on a 'good front' and conceal the fact that they are struggling to understand or keep up with what is going on.

If the person was used to partaking in more complex activities, it may be the case that these become too hard for the person to follow and family and friends may need to tactfully suggest to the person that they might find it more satisfying to take up something less demanding. The person may of course need to be assisted with making the switch to another activity.

Language and communication difficulties may also start to emerge. At this phase the person is likely to retain the ability to understand language and will know what others are saying to them, but their ability to respond appropriately may start to be compromised – in particular, they may find it hard to recall the names of things and sometimes muddle up sentences. Patience is required on the part of those conversing with the person. We may need to give them extra time to get their message across or to tactfully ask them to repeat the message.

Another thing that can try the patience of families and friends is the tendency for some people with early dementia to become very repetitive in what they say, sometimes repeating the same thing many times in a conversation, or including the same messages in each conversation they have. We must realise that this comes from the person's memory difficulties, specifically their forgetting that they have said the same thing before (we will discuss these matters further in Chapter 4).

We may also notice the person's manner or behaviour starts to change – as we discussed in Chapter 2 this is often the first sign of young-onset dementia. Sometimes the person may become more touchy, anxious, rude or even aggressive and family and friends must adopt a calm and unprovoking manner. Tact and skilful communication will help resolve potentially problematic situations.

> 'One of the daft arguments we have with Grandma is about getting her to the hairdressers; my mum's very keen that she keeps up with that so we take her every week. Sometimes when we go round, for no reason at all she'll shout "I'm not going" and that's not the grandma I remember. I tend to make a joke of it where I can – one thing Grandma is good at talking about is the weather, we have a lot of conversations about the weather and normally over and over again, so I say to her, "Next week it might be raining and we might not want to go then so we really should go this week."'

More often the person may appear more vacant or detached than before and sometimes rather self-absorbed and less interested in other people. This is a sign that their ability to understand and manage all the complexities of their social world is starting to become impaired: their memory and attention difficulties meaning that they find it increasingly hard to cope with the range of people, events, messages, sights and sounds that we are all bombarded with all the time. We should recognise the need to avoid over-stimulating the person – for example, by inviting them for a meal with just one or two other people rather than a large party.

It is also possible that the person may be experiencing depression – up to a quarter of people with dementia may become depressed at some time during their illness. We should not be afraid to ask the person how they are feeling and help them get medical assistance if necessary. People with dementia can get over depression by talking about their feelings, or through receiving counselling or anti-depressant drugs.

ACCEPTANCE

This is our final key principle for family members and friends of a person with early dementia. We need to learn to accept the person's changing abilities, manner and behaviour if they are to remain socially included. We have already mentioned qualities such as patience, tact and having an unprovoking manner when interacting with the person on a day-to-day basis. We must accept that repetition, forgetfulness, self-absorption and other challenges are all part of the person's growing difficulties, and we must learn to adapt to them and live with them.

> 'The outreach worker was very helpful. She was the person who advised me to "go with the flow" however bizarre it seems. She said, "Who is the problem for, is it for your husband or is it for you?" and if the problem is for you just let it go.'

> 'Give people time; let them do things in their own way and don't take over if it hasn't been done "properly". You need to learn to ask yourself does it really matter?'

It is also important that we learn to accept that a person is changing and that we need to adapt our view of them accordingly. This can be hard for some family members and friends to do. For example, Mike was a successful businessman, but now has dementia. He attends a day centre regularly, but believes that when the transport comes to take him there he is going to a business meeting and insists on taking his briefcase and a notebook with him. This upsets Mike's wife Mary, who tries to stop him from doing so – 'you don't need that where you're going,' she says. This in turn upsets Mike. Dementia empathy implies that we should try to appreciate how the person with dementia understands and manages their social world, and accept that their way of doing so is an appropriate response to their changing situation. Surely it would be better for Mary to accept that this is how Mike understands and copes with his situation, and to let him take his briefcase if he wants to.

> 'I think my mum feels a huge responsibility for Grandma, being an only child. She drives herself crazy worrying about what Grandma's eating and I know her diet's not ideal but she's happy… I don't think it's worth having the argument with her over something you can't change. It's about being as patient as you can and picking your fights as the saying goes. My mum has a tendency to pick up on everything with my grandma and I just don't see the point of that as it puts her in a bad mood and stresses you out.'

Accepting that the person is changing can also help us to resist the urge to avoid them because 'it isn't really her'. In some ways that might be true, in that their behaviour and outlook may have changed, but ultimately it is her (or him) – the mother, father, aunt, uncle, husband, wife or friend that we have always known and loved.

Another aspect of acceptance is that family members and friends may need to help the person be accepted by others who may not have the same level of understanding or tolerance of people with dementia. We have talked about the stigma that society may display towards people with dementia and the negative stereotype of dementia that can sometimes be expressed in the media. There may be people within the person's family or circle of friends who find it hard to accept that the person should continue to be part of social occasions or activities. We can help by providing a good example of acceptance, or sometimes by tactfully offering information about dementia to those whose understanding may not be as complete as ours.

> 'I think a couple of our neighbours have found it quite difficult. My husband sometimes says things that are inappropriate due to the nature of his dementia and he must have said something rude to a neighbour. One day he avoided us both in the street; he had previously ignored my husband but not me. I wrote to him explaining the reason but have not heard anything back from him. It's been very upsetting.'

> 'Sometimes in the evening they'd wander to the local pub and they'd have a drink, just one and then wander back and people in the local community always said, "Oh your dad was marvellous with your mum" and they would make a fuss of my mum and that was good for Dad, it got him out of the house and my mum would respond. Even when she didn't have any conversation she would smile at people – for him it was trying to keep a bit of normality in the changing situation.'

Compiling a life story

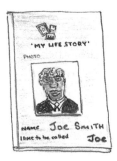

This is a very practical way that family members and friends may support a person in the early phase of dementia and assist them to prepare for the future. It is exactly what it sounds like: a history or story of the person's life to date. The resulting life story could take many forms; many are in the form of books filled with photographs, written accounts, letters, certificates and so on that together tell the story of the person's life. Some people use digital media when putting together a life history, compiling photograph shows or videos. Life story albums are also being developed on social media internet sites such as Facebook.

Life stories can be compiled by family members, friends or professional carers at any time during a person's journey through dementia, but there is a clear advantage of compiling one during the early phase, when the person themselves can contribute to deciding what goes into them and can appreciate the result. Life stories are valuable in a number of ways:

- They provide a point of reference for people with dementia themselves. As their condition progresses and they start to forget aspects of their past lives, they can look at their life story to remind themselves of the person they have been.

- Family members and friends can also use a life story as a reminder about the person they once knew as they see that person slowly changing.

- If in the future the person attends a day centre or care home, staff will find a life story invaluable for becoming better acquainted with the person as a person, and will be able to see them as an individual with a rich past. It may also help them understand the person's manner and behaviour better if they can relate that behaviour to aspects of the person's past life (see Chapters 5 and 6).

As stated earlier, if compiled in the early phase of dementia when the person still has some awareness, the person can contribute and decide themselves what goes into it and what is left out. There may of course be particular aspects of their life that the person would prefer to be left unrecorded, such as events that were upsetting or that have been kept secret. It does not matter if a life story is not complete; more important is that it reflects and celebrates the person's life. Written biographies are always selective, presenting the person in a particular way, and there is no reason why a life story should be any different.

Intimacy and sexuality

Many people with early dementia live with their spouse or partner and will have been used to intimate and sexual relationships. Frequently sexual relationships continue into old age. The question then arises: what should happen to intimacy and sexual relationships if one partner develops dementia?

If a person retains awareness and mental capacity, there should not be an issue because they have the ability to consent to sexual relationships and those relationships can continue as before. But what if the person's awareness of their condition seems to be declining and their capacity to make decisions is compromised? Let us consider an example of a married couple who have always enjoyed sex. The wife develops dementia but retains awareness in the early phase and still participates willingly in sexual activities. But then dementia progresses and she lacks the capacity to make decisions in most situations. However, she still responds positively when her husband makes sexual overtures towards her, they continue to have sex and she seems to enjoy it. Is this right, or might her husband be sexually exploiting or even abusing her?

We would argue that this does not have to be the case. Ethicists suggest that, even if a person cannot give consent to an activity in the strict sense of the word, they can still display willingness to participate in it and we can gauge that willingness by their actions, words and mood – if they actually take part in the activity, say they are enjoying it and appear content and happy, then we may assume they are willing to do it. As we will see in subsequent chapters, the principle of willingness provides the basis for carrying out a whole range of social and recreational activities with people with more advanced dementia, and we believe it can equally apply to our husband and wife's sexual activities – we can assume that she is willing because of her actions, words and mood, and because they match how she has always responded to her husband's sexual advances.

The situation becomes more complex if, as sometimes happens, the onset of dementia leads to a change in a person's level of interest in sexual activities. If they become less interested, then their partner should respect that – dementia empathy means that we need to appreciate that the change derives from the person's dementia and we should accept and adapt to that change. If the person's level of interest increases, problems can arise if their partner does not wish to have more sex and within the relationship the situation will have to be resolved the best way it can be – whether or not a person in a relationship has dementia, sex should only take place within that relationship if both partners are willing for it to happen.

More challenging still is the case where dementia leads to the person making sexual overtures towards others. If the person is unattached and the individual that they make advances to is attracted to the person, is it right for them to respond? Would the principle of willingness apply in this case? We are not so sure – the potential for exploitation and abuse is perhaps too great. Also, suppose for a moment that the person is suddenly cured of their dementia and is told how they have been acting. The chances are that they would be embarrassed, ashamed or horrified. In some cases it is more appropriate for us to adopt a 'paternalistic' approach towards people with dementia when their behaviour may cause distress to others, or would cause themselves distress if they became aware of what they were doing.

> 'I would really like to talk to someone about sexual relations. It's a big hole in the literature and seems to get glossed over. I don't know how to approach it, as it was an important part of our relationship. I try to find ways of staying intimate but sometimes this doesn't work which feels like another loss.'

Maintaining and giving up independence in the early phase of dementia

At the onset of dementia a person will of course be more or less independent. They may be living on their own and will be able to look after themselves and carry out activities on their own. We have stated previously that a key aim of supporting a person with dementia is for them to maintain independence as much as possible for as long as possible, and we have set out the benefits of being independent. In this section we will consider some more specific ways that family members and friends can assist a person with early dementia to maintain independence, and the sometimes difficult situations that can arise when independence needs to be given up.

> 'My wife used to go for a walk around the village but she was beginning to get lost so I had started to follow her. I had told people in the village by this time so people knew there was a problem.'

ASSISTIVE TECHNOLOGY

We have considered previously ways that a person may be assisted to compensate for increasing memory loss and difficulties in completing complex tasks through the use of lists, reminders, labels and clearly set out instructions. All these strategies will of course enhance their ability to remain independent. In the early phase, when the person retains awareness, they may well be able to devise their own memory-supporting strategies. To complement such approaches, the concept of assistive technology has been developed. This is the use of both low- and high-tech devices to help people remain independent and reduce the risks of their coming to harm. Assistive technology is not new – anyone who wears spectacles, has a hearing aid or a walking stick, is using assistive technology. Slightly more sophisticated are items such as calendar clocks that display the date as well as the time, which some people with dementia find useful for keeping track of days of the week. We have previously mentioned mobile phones as useful aids for a person to keep in touch with family and friends, offering the opportunity of giving them quick reminders through text messaging or enabling them to phone someone if they get into difficulties when out of the house.

Some more specialised technological aids are available for people with early dementia. Examples include computerised reminders, such as a device that gives a person a message when they are about to leave the house to remember to take their door key. Safety technology includes heat or flood detectors, or devices that automatically switch off gas taps if someone leaves them on. Leisure devices include easy-to-use radios and music players. Another potential benefit of assistive technology is the use of tracking devices that are worn by the person with dementia and use GPS technology so that their whereabouts can be known at all times. Such technology may allow them to go out on their own and be 'found' if they get lost.

Yet another new development is the increased interest of some health and social care authorities in establishing support based on electronic devices that are placed around a person's house to monitor anything that may compromise their safety, such as gas leaks, floods, fire or if they have fallen or gone out of the house unexpectedly. These devices are connected to a central monitoring point and alarms are raised if the system reports anything untoward.

Assistive technology has clear benefits if it is successful in assisting a person to live independently and safely, and its use can offer considerable reassurance to family and friends. However, it is not a panacea and a number of drawbacks have been identified:

- It can work for some people but not others; for example, one person may understand and respond to computerised reminders while another may be more confused by them. All technology is complex and dementia may quickly compromise a person's ability to relate to it.

- Assistive technology devices can be expensive and may not be freely available from the government.

- There has been some debate about the use of tracking aids because of concern that they may compromise privacy and human rights. However, it is also considered that they can help support risk assessment and discussions with people with dementia indicate that their use is felt to be in their best interests and not an infringement of their rights. Most importantly, any decision about using such devices should be taken based on knowing the person, thinking about their capacity and balancing risks with independence. It is possible that a person could give permission for such devices to be used as part of an advanced decision.

Assistive technologies can bring great reassurance to families and friends that someone is safe, especially when they are not nearby. However, they should not be seen as a replacement for social contact.

DRIVING

This is an aspect of daily life that can create considerable anxiety for family members and friends. There is no intrinsic reason why a person with early dementia cannot continue to drive if they retain awareness and ability – a diagnosis of dementia does not automatically exclude a person from having a driving licence in countries such as the UK, though the diagnosis would have to be declared to insurers. However, the progression of dementia will inevitably compromise the person's ability to drive safely. Growing memory loss can lead to difficulty remembering routes or interpreting road signs. Attention deficits will affect the person's ability to concentrate on the road and notice potential hazards, and executive function impairment will compromise their ability to make appropriate decisions while driving. Sometimes a person with dementia can continue to drive for a while if someone is with them to give directions and point out hazards, but sooner or later the point is reached when it is realised that they could harm themselves or others if they continue to attempt to drive.

> 'My husband would drive along in low gears or wouldn't change
> down gears and didn't understand why the car was juddering.
> We'd have to tell him to change gear.'

Giving up driving can be traumatic for a person and for their families and friends. Sometimes they realise themselves that they can't cope at the wheel and give up driving voluntarily, or acquiesce to family members' entreaties that they should not drive.

> 'My husband drove to a nearby town which is only a seven
> mile journey that he had done for 30 years, and couldn't find
> his way home. He came home having driven around for three
> hours, unable to find a single landmark that he recognised. He
> came in in a cold sweat, and threw the keys on the table saying:
> "Never let me drive again!"'

But in some cases driving is brought to an end by a person having an accident or being stopped by the police and their licence taken away after a driving assessment. Other people with dementia lack awareness that their driving abilities are no longer acceptable and refuse to give up driving. How should families respond in such cases?

Some family members in these circumstances resort to acts of deception to prevent the person driving. They may hide the car keys and pretend to the person that they have been lost. They may remove the battery leads so that the car cannot start or they may sell the car, telling the person it has been written off in an accident. Is it right to use deceptions such as these with people with dementia? Some would say that deception in any circumstance is ethically wrong: it dehumanises the person and, if they find out they have been lied to, it can make the situation worse. On the other hand, some would feel that deception in this situation is worth it to prevent the person harming themselves or others by continuing to drive. They would point out that deception is a fact of life – how often do we tell half-truths or white lies or keep things to ourselves as part of our everyday relationships with others? We will consider the role of deception in dementia care further in Chapter 4.

WHERE SHOULD A PERSON WITH EARLY DEMENTIA LIVE?

Many people with dementia who live in 'the community' live with their spouse, who is most likely to take on the main caring role. With dementia affecting in the main people at the older end of the age spectrum, the person's spouse is likely to be themselves elderly. Others live with their adult children – who may well be in their 50s, 60s or older – and a significant number live alone. This is likely to reflect their own preference and they may well manage effectively in their own familiar surroundings, with the support of family and friends. We have already discussed strategies and aids for helping a person with dementia maintain independence and, while these do not apply exclusively to people with dementia who live alone, they clearly have considerable potential value to those people. But what if dementia has progressed to the point where despite such supports the person may be at risk of harm from neglect, accident or possible exploitation?

Part of the answer may be enhanced professional support that can help the person remain in their own home (see later). But sooner or later a specific question may arise for a relative or close friend of a person with dementia.

SHOULD MY RELATIVE OR FRIEND COME TO LIVE WITH ME?

It may seem obvious that a person with early dementia who finds it difficult to live alone but who does not need or want residential care should go to live with a close relative or friend, especially when it is a son or daughter, and this is what many people do. However, it is not a decision to be taken lightly and families considering such a move have many factors to weigh up in coming to that decision. First, is it what the person with dementia wants? Many would find such a move comforting and would enjoy the company, but some would prefer not to burden others or would find life in a younger family noisy and difficult. Second, is the family prepared for the extra burden and potential stress of having a person with dementia in the household, even if it is a loved parent? Research shows that adult children caring for a person with dementia in their household experience more stress than other carers. It can change their lives: adult children may find themselves having to give up work in order to look after their parent – caring for a person with dementia can have greater financial implications than other forms of caring. Previously difficult family relationships may resurface leading to conflict, and if the adult child has their own children still at home they might be torn between their needs and the needs of their parent.

Alternatively there can be many positives for families and friends in taking people into their own homes, such as maintaining relationships, giving something back and gaining satisfaction from the caring role. However, the stresses are very real and it is important that decisions to make such arrangements are thought through very carefully. Possible alternatives such as supported accommodation or paid care at home should also be considered with the person before making a decision.

Health and social care support for people with early dementia, their families and friends

As we suggested in the previous chapter, professional support for people with early dementia can sometimes be thin on the ground. Once the person has received a diagnosis, unless they are taking ACEI drugs, they are likely to receive limited offers of professional help and simply be told to contact their GP if and when problems occur. Financial limitations mean that local authorities concentrate their resources on those further through the dementia journey who are deemed to have greater need. Thus begins what we call the 'gap years' when families and friends are often left supporting people with early dementia with little or no professional help. Another issue for families and friends is that provision can be very variable in different places, leading to frustration when a service or facility may be available for some but not for others.

So what may be available during the 'gap years'? The following are the main areas of help that may be accessed. The 'Resources for Family and Friends' section at the end of this book lists organisations, websites and other available resources in English-speaking countries.

SUPPORT GROUPS

Groups of family members and friends of people with dementia may come together, often facilitated by voluntary sector organisations, in order to meet each other, share experiences and help each other out. Some support groups have separate get-togethers for people with dementia themselves while their carers are having their own meetings. Sometimes invited speakers attend to give talks on important topics. Support groups are not to everyone's taste and some people may have practical problems with attending meetings but many find being in touch with a local support group invaluable.

> 'I think I have managed to feel a bit more assertive and confident through support from Uniting Carers for Dementia UK. I been able to stand up for myself and in getting my husband's needs addressed. Having contact with other carers and feeling that I have rights as a carer, it's important to stick together.'

INTERNET SITES

Charities and other bodies have extensive websites packed with information and advice. These websites often also include forums or chat rooms where those supporting a person with dementia – and sometimes people with dementia themselves – can communicate online with others.

> 'I recently used the Alzheimer's Society talking point and it was useful to find out how other people cope with difficult situations; it was quite reassuring.'

ADVICE AND SIGNPOSTING SERVICES

In some countries steps are being taken to set up services that people in the early phase of dementia and their families may contact for advice and signposting to other sources of professional help. Advice services have links to health and social services and can make it easier for families to access such services if difficulties arise. Provision of such services is, however, very limited at present and in some areas may not be available at all.

DAY CENTRES

As the name suggests, these are facilities that people with dementia can attend during the working day, to be looked after while family members have a rest or go to work and where they can take part in activities and socialise with others. Many family members find the respite that day centres provide invaluable and many people with dementia enjoy attending them. However, not all people with dementia relish day centres – if a person has been reserved and private throughout their life, they may not find being with other people easy. The best day centres have a wide range of activities and staff who understand the needs of those who attend and offer advice and support to family members.

> 'I think the first time they needed help was when Mum started to not settle at night and Dad would say he was tired and that's when we looked into Mum going to the day centre.'

> 'They have offered my grandma the chance to go to community centres and things but she's not a joiner-in, she never has been and we couldn't expect her to do it now.'

> 'My husband attends a day centre two days per week and this allows me to have some time for myself and to keep on top of things. It also gives him some independence and space away from me...a little bit of life outside of my control.'

HOME CARE

If a person has been assessed as requiring assistance with aspects of their physical health or daily living care, care at home can be provided to help them with such things as getting bathed and dressed or at mealtimes. Provision of home care can be very variable with some authorities offering more than others, and the extent that people with dementia may have to pay for such care may also vary from area to area. While many home carers are skilled and committed, the quality of home care has been criticised, with complaints that visits are extremely brief, with staff given strict limits on how long they should spend with a person and often lack of consistency of staff, with different workers attending each day so that no one actually gets to know the person with dementia.

> 'We've had some really lovely carers who genuinely do really nice things for my grandma and that really helps…it's nice when you can feel you can trust people.'

> 'Introducing a home carer was very difficult as my wife didn't want any help; the first person didn't work as my wife didn't like her. However when Jane started it worked well from the beginning. She was very skilled and did things like going shopping with my wife, made her feel included. This was such a relief. It took a few weeks before they settled in but eventually my wife thought Jane was lovely.'

PERSONAL ASSISTANTS AND PRIVATE CARERS

Sometimes families directly employ people to provide care and in some countries the government may provide a personalised care budget that the family can spend as they wish. They may employ professional carers from an agency, which helps to ensure liability and protection, or some people may choose to employ a friend or neighbour directly to offer care. There can be great advantages in being able to choose the right person and in ensuring continuity of carers, but it is also important that advice is sought about how to protect the person receiving care who may be vulnerable. In addition, managing a budget can also be difficult for people in early phases of dementia or family members, so this should be thought through carefully.

> 'I arranged for one day a week replacement care at home to give me a break, and sometimes I had a stretch of five

consecutive days. It was always the same person who was employed to come in. Without those breaks I don't think I could have made it.'

SUPPORTED ACCOMMODATION

As a compromise between living alone and entering residential care, some people with dementia live in supported accommodation. This means that they have their own flat or apartment and live more or less independently, but staff are available on site for some or all of the day to ensure that residents are managing and to assist if necessary.

24-HOUR RESPITE CARE

Forms of respite care other than day or home care may be available to enable a person's main carer to take a break. Sometimes it can be arranged for someone to stay with the person while the carer goes away for a holiday – other family members or friends may of course take on this role, or a paid carer may be employed. Alternatively, a person with dementia may themselves spend a week or two in a care home while their carer has a break. Again, paying for respite care may be an issue and the change of environment as well as quality of care are important considerations (see Chapter 6).

THE 'GAP YEARS' – A FALSE ECONOMY?

Research is increasingly suggesting that minimising support services during the 'gap years' of early dementia because of financial constraints may be a false economy, because people with dementia and their families who receive particular forms of support or input may do better than those who do not, with the person maybe progressing through dementia at a slower rate and families being able to manage caring for the person for longer. Specific interventions that have been shown by research to have such benefits but are only infrequently available include the following.

- Psycho-social interventions: carried out by community mental health practitioners, these include specific education, counselling and stress management techniques aiming to improve family members' ability to care for the person with dementia and enhance their emotional coping resources; they may reduce rates of admission to residential care.

- Cognitive stimulation techniques for people in the early phase of dementia: sometimes carried out individually with the person and sometimes within group sessions, according to some research, these may be as good as or better than ACEI drugs in slowing the progression of dementia and they may also improve a person's mood.

Families and friends sometimes feel that they have been left to their own devices and that more information and support in the early phase of dementia may have eased the journey in the later phases. We may help by supporting campaigns that are seeking to improve the provision of professional support available for those in the early phase of dementia.

> 'You need to have someone who can co-ordinate things for you and who understands the system…someone to talk to – a point of contact who knows about what you are going through and understands your situation.'

> 'I would have liked one person I could have contacted – someone who doesn't just say I can deal with one bit of it and that someone else deals with the other bits.'

Family members and friends: looking after oneself and each other

It will be clear from what we have said that being a family member or friend of someone with early dementia will place emotional and sometimes practical demands on an individual and will require considerable personal skills and qualities. As we have observed, a comparison might be made with becoming a new parent – it is a demanding role for which few people have been given any preparation or training and which will carry continual responsibility for a considerable period of time. A key difference with parenthood that may well increase the subjective demands on someone supporting a person with dementia is that most new parents have chosen to have children and welcome the role. This is not usually the case with dementia. Looking after oneself and each other is crucial for maintaining well-being for both supporters and people with dementia alike.

> 'I never thought of myself as a carer; it wasn't a profession I ever wanted or was trained for. I worked with children with special needs but it's different when it's in your personal life.'

> 'In the great scheme of dementia my grandma's not too bad but everyone's perceptions are different and the worst thing that's happened to you is the worst thing in the world.'

> 'So my husband and I both had to give up work, and that was one year after diagnosis. That meant an enormous drop in finances; teachers' pensions are generous but between us we missed out on 25 years of service and therefore the pension was much smaller. I reckon we lost over a million pounds of earnings by not being able to work until we were 60 or 65.'

There is little 'rocket science' behind the principles of looking after oneself. Supporters of people with dementia cope with the demands placed on them in the same way that they have become accustomed to coping with other demands throughout their lives. Everyone has their own way of managing situations and emotional demands and it is often a matter of recognising that one is in need of emotional refreshment and reaching for one's familiar coping strategies. Key principles of personal and mutual support include the following.

- Talking with others: having an outlet for one's feelings, thoughts and anxieties is always useful. Being able to talk about one's situation with trusted family members or friends will help keep that situation in perspective.

Alternatively, support groups or internet forums may provide opportunities to talk with others in similar positions.

'I have been lucky as I've had a really good friend; we have just talked for hours and hours.'

- Being available to others: as we have been saying, it is important that family members and friends do not avoid contact with the person with dementia or with their main supporter. Sharing the supporting role makes that role easier and being able to interact with a range of family members and friends will help enhance the quality of life of the person with dementia.

'It all started with a good friend over the road who walked a dog. He said, "Do you think your husband will come round the village with me when I walk the dog?" So I said, "Let's try it." And this is how it began. Then other dog walkers and habitual strollers met them on their rounds, and people in the village formed a rota to accompany my husband on his walk every day – enabling him to enjoy the fresh air and me to have a bit of respite from the constant vigilance.'

- Recognising stressors: supporters need a good measure of self-awareness, to recognise when their feelings of anxiety or burden are becoming too much. It is important to acknowledge that there will be times when one feels under pressure. It is also important to recognise that we are not superheroes – we cannot do everything or get everything right, we can only do what we can.

'I had to ask the GP what to do as I was a bit at my wits' end.'

- Taking time out: it can be tiring and sometimes frustrating being with a person with dementia for an extended period of time. Often the person has continual needs and anxieties and may follow one around, sometimes asking the same questions many times. Using the principles of dementia empathy, we can recognise that this reflects their uncertainty about themselves due to their memory loss and lack of ability to orientate themselves to what is happening around them. But we may still become frustrated with the person and this frustration could boil over. Better to take 'time out' from the person, have a cup of tea and let our feelings subside.

'I sometimes need to just walk into a different room and have a breather as I can feel myself getting cross and that doesn't help.'

- Taking breaks and holidays: if one is a full-time supporter of a person with dementia, one should try to give oneself regular breaks and holidays. Friends and other family members could assist by volunteering to stay with the person while their main supporter goes out for the evening or takes a holiday. Support services such as day centres or respite care may be employed. It is a good idea if one is on a respite break to avoid the temptation felt by many supporters of people with dementia to continually check that the person is all right, by phoning the respite facility or even visiting the person there – a break should be a break.

'Having time for me was really helpful; having time to do something different; being able to do what I wanted to do.'

- Keeping up with hobbies and interests: breaks and respite periods may of course be used for supporters' own hobbies and interests and it is important that supporters make time during the day for things they like to do.

'Dad played bowls a lot and he enjoyed it and it was a bit of time for himself. We didn't want Dad to give up his bowling so during the bowling season we would between us have Mum with us so she had someone with her.'

- Understanding the nature of dementia: the more we know about dementia the better we can understand a person's manner and behaviour and the more effectively we can interact with and support the person. Also, having explanations for the person's manner can help us recognise the reasons why they are acting that way, which may help reduce the stress that such behaviour may provoke.

'I would have liked more information because at this point you don't need services but you need information in order to support the person with dementia better.'

'I could have done with someone earlier to talk with me about "bossiness", not taking over and scolding, and doing *with* rather than *for*.'

- Using support services: as we have said, support services can sometimes appear to be thin on the ground during the early phase of dementia, but it is important that supporters know how to access them.

'I think I would benefit from having time to deal with my emotions; I tend to hide from it all and then collapse in a heap. I get very angry with my husband sometimes and I know I shouldn't but it makes me feel bad. If I could work these things through with someone, I think it would help us both.'

CHAPTER 4

More Help Needed

The Phase of Moderate Dementia

The characteristics of moderate dementia

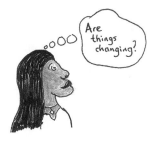

It can of course be hard to say when a person moves from the early to moderate phase of dementia. These are not discrete stages and people may have some symptoms and not others. Some people may remain in the earlier phase of dementia for quite a few years and with the right support can maintain relative independence. This is particularly apparent for those who have been given a diagnosis at an early stage. For others the progression of the illness appears more marked, especially if given a diagnosis at a later stage, and a noticeable decline in function may be observed. Broadly speaking, a person with symptoms of moderate dementia will display some characteristic difficulties. These may be present regardless of the actual type of dementia because by this phase most forms of dementia are beginning to share similarities.

- Memory problems will be more profound and the person will have increased difficulty in remembering new information. Memories of their past life may begin to be impaired. Some things may be forgotten completely while other things may become muddled or half remembered. This can lead to the person believing things that are not now the case, such as that they are still going to work or that a long-dead relative is still alive.

- The person may have lost awareness of their condition and have limited understanding that there is anything amiss.

- The person is likely to have problems with understanding complex concepts. They may be unable to read any more than simple sentences, and hobbies or activities that involve complex reasoning, such as many card games, quizzes or crosswords, may be too difficult.

- The person's orientation to their surroundings often becomes more impaired. They may have problems with finding their way around safely in unfamiliar surroundings or with understanding the time or date and not know what season of the year it is. They will usually still recognise significant people, such as family members and friends, but may not remember or recognise less familiar others.

- For some people language abilities may become more impaired. If this happens, sentence construction can be compromised and the person may have increased difficulty with word finding. While they should still be able to understand what others say to them so long as the message isn't too complex, they may well have difficulty in making a coherent reply. Often the content of what they say may be limited to simple ideas and be repetitive.

- The person's ability to attend to events or concentrate for long periods will be compromised. Their interest in other people may appear to reduce, though this is more to do with memory, comprehension and attention difficulties than evidence of the person becoming more self-centred.

- Changes in personality or manner may become apparent and tend to be expressed through behaviour. Some people become very passive and withdrawn while others appear restless and agitated at times and may be prone to aggressive outbursts that do not appear to have a cause. Some people appear to have a great need for physical activity and walking about. People may also say things or behave in a way that appears hurtful or insensitive. This can be particularly difficult for close family or friends and will be addressed in more detail in Chapter 5.

- The person is likely to begin to find daily living activities more difficult. They may have problems preparing meals or drinks for themselves. Most people will still be able to eat and drink without assistance although preferences for food may change – for example, they may come to prefer sweeter or spicy food. They are likely still to be able to wash and dress themselves but may get muddled, putting clothes on in the wrong order or forgetting particular things. They may begin to have difficulties with using the toilet, leading to occasional accidents.

- Unless they have unrelated physical health problems, the person is still likely to be physically well and active and can usually get about without assistance other than finding their way in unfamiliar places. However, for some people who have visual-perceptual difficulties, there may be problems with recognising and interpreting their environment. For example, patterns on floors, poor lighting, mirrors, ill-defined contrasts between walls and doors may cause the person difficulties with moving about.

In short, the person is likely to exhibit increased levels of 'confusion', which in Chapter 1 we explained in terms of their having problems in either understanding the world around them, or being able to respond appropriately to the world around them, or both. As with the early phase of dementia, appreciating the specific difficulties that the person has and trying to see the world the way they see it – dementia empathy – will help us interact with and support them more effectively.

Where do people with moderate dementia live?

By this phase, most people will struggle to live on their own, unless they have intensive support from family members, friends or professionals. More likely they will be living with a main carer, often a spouse, partner or adult child. Some may be able to live in 'sheltered accommodation' with on-site professional support. Some families may by this time be considering residential care for the person or that transition may have been made. We will consider the issues around residential care in Chapter 6. For now, we will make no assumptions about where the person with moderate dementia is living, but will consider aspects of social and interpersonal support that family members and friends may apply in any setting. The principles we discuss are equally valuable for professional care staff in settings such as day centres, sheltered accommodation or care homes.

The changing nature of relationships

Family members and friends will become acutely aware of the fact that their relationship with the person is changing, with that relationship becoming increasingly less equal as the person's condition progresses.

> 'It feels like my husband's disappearing – for example, he says things that are not in character. It's losing someone: I feel like I'm being widowed before he's gone. It's like living with someone that you don't know, but at other times I get a reminder of our closeness.'

Moderate dementia will clearly place more responsibility on the person's supporters. At the same time, the person will find it harder to respond to others as they used to. They may appear less interested in other people's lives or concerns and may be less able to show or reciprocate affection. They will by now have noticeably changed and it can be harder for family members and friends to recognise them as they once were, particularly regarding their cognitive abilities and sometimes their behaviour and manner as well.

> 'She changed enormously and this was the most difficult thing to cope with; I wasn't able to share decisions and it begins to feel like you are looking after a stranger.'

These changes may be distressing for families and friends. Many will feel an acute sense of loss, of the person they once knew – the progression of dementia has sometimes been called a 'living bereavement' for those close to the person. The temptation to avoid the person may become great for those not obliged to directly care for them and friends may become increasingly distant especially if behaviour changes. For the person who has dementia, social situations can become difficult to cope with and they may become distressed or want to avoid them.

> 'Slowly all our friends were disappearing; our social circle was diminishing. Only close friends were allowed in the house.'

> 'As time has gone on it's made a lot of difference to social relations. We have a lot of friends who don't find it easy especially as my husband's behaviour has become more difficult. Some friends and neighbours have drifted away.'

Those who have adopted the role of main carer will feel most profoundly the change in the nature of their relationship with the person. A spouse or long-term partner, who was used to an equal relationship of mutual interdependence, will have to come to terms with the person with dementia depending on them. An adult child, who may have relied to an extent on their parent for support and help throughout their life, may now have to provide that support and help themselves. There is no easy way for family members and friends to come to terms with the relationship changes that come with the progression of dementia. Above all it is important to accept that the person has changed and, while we can still recognise aspects of them as the person they were and hold onto these, we also need to accept the differences that dementia can bring.

Mutual support remains crucial, as does trying to maintain an attitude of wanting the best for the person and helping them to lead as satisfying a life as possible. For family members or friends who are providing direct care, it is essential to accept support from others both practically and emotionally, especially as the needs of the person with dementia become greater. The temptation may be to 'soldier on' and try to cope, because it can be difficult to ask for help, but it is really important to look after your own needs and share the caring.

> 'It was helpful having someone who could say to me, "This is what you need to do."'

> 'Other friends have become closer and offer to sit with my husband and that's really important.'

The person's growing difficulties also mean that family members and friends must learn to interact with them in a new way. This may be represented diagrammatically. Normal relationships can be expressed in this simple form:

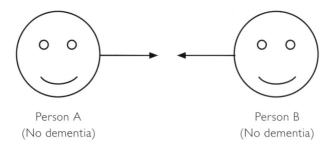

Person A
(No dementia)

Person B
(No dementia)

When both people have similar abilities, their communication is equal and reciprocal – both can reach out to each other and expect a response. But now consider a relationship between Person A and Person C, who has difficulties as a result of moderate dementia:

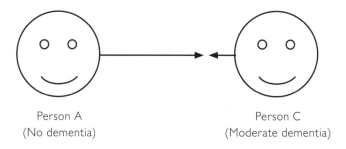

Person A
(No dementia)

Person C
(Moderate dementia)

People with moderate dementia cannot reach out to others in the same way. This means that Person A must make more effort to reach out and have a relationship with Person C. This may be reflected in the way that Person A interacts with Person C. The British psychologist Tom Kitwood (1997, p.89) expressed it thus: 'The quality of interaction is warmer, richer in feeling, than that of everyday life.'

Communication and language in moderate dementia

Human relationships are expressed through communication and language and it is with impairments in a person's ability to communicate effectively that the changes of moderate dementia are most evident. Learning to understand what a person with moderate dementia is trying to communicate and knowing how best to respond to them is a key task for family members and friends.

Language is of course central to communication, but communication is more than just language. Much of our communication with others is done non-verbally, through our expression, manner and actions. This is even more the case with a person with moderate dementia, whose verbal language abilities may be compromised. As we will see in Chapter 5, much of the behaviour of people with dementia that others find difficult is likely to represent their attempts to communicate non-verbally needs and wishes that they cannot express through language.

LANGUAGE DIFFICULTIES IN MODERATE DEMENTIA

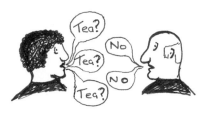

A person's language and communication difficulties will largely reflect the more global difficulties of moderate dementia. As memory deficits and decline of cognitive abilities become more profound, the person may say less or their conversation may include muddled memories or become very repetitive. Also, they may not understand abstract ideas and can mistake the person talking to them with someone else, perhaps a significant family member from the past. Growing attention issues make it hard for them to concentrate on what others are saying to them, and impairment of executive function may mean that they struggle to follow even simple instructions. Sometimes they may appear to be talking to someone, which can be as a result of visual hallucinations – seeing people or things that are not there. They may also display difficulties with communication that reflect damage to the language areas of the brain, such as word-finding problems. For some people who have a particular type of dementia called 'semantic dementia', which affects the temporal lobes of the brain, specific problems include remembering the meaning of words, faces and objects. The person may know what they want to say but cannot put their message into a coherent form – we tend to label what they are saying as 'rambling' or 'confused' talk, but it clearly means something to the person concerned. Sometimes they display *perseveration*, a tendency to repeat the same word or phrase over and over, like a stuck record. Understanding what may be behind the person's language difficulties is the first step to becoming able to communicate with them effectively.

HOW *NOT* TO COMMUNICATE WITH A
PERSON WITH MODERATE DEMENTIA

There are many mistakes we can make when communicating with people with moderate dementia. These mistakes matter, because if the person perceives them they can increase their sense of ill-being or lack of worth. The British psychologist Tom Kitwood (1997) researched into this area and identified common communication errors that he termed 'malignant social psychology'. His research was carried out with professional care staff, but family members and friends may well recognise in Kitwood's categories some of their own ways of interacting – the following is not a complete list:

Infantilisation	Addressing a person very patronisingly, as an insensitive person might treat a young child.
Outpacing	Providing information, presenting choices, etc. at a rate too fast for the person to understand; putting them under pressure to do things more rapidly than they can bear.
Ignoring	Carrying on a conversation in the presence of a person as if they were not there.
Accusation	Blaming a person for actions or failures of action that arise from their lack of ability, or their misunderstanding of the situation.
Mockery	Making fun of the person's 'strange' actions or remarks; teasing, humiliating, making jokes at their expense.
Disparagement	Telling a person they are incompetent, useless, worthless or otherwise giving them messages that are damaging to their self-esteem.

(Kitwood 1997, p.46)

How many of these communication errors did you recognise and, if you are honest, have found yourself making – or heard others make? We have observed earlier that people with moderate dementia may well retain the ability to understand what is said to them, at least at a simple level, long after their ability to communicate verbally themselves has been lost and, if a person heard and understood a family member or friend communicating in these ways, it would clearly upset them, even if they could not always express that upset.

LISTENING AND RESPONDING TO A PERSON WITH MODERATE DEMENTIA

People with moderate dementia want to talk and interact, and family members and friends should encourage them to do so. To the extent that their communications are understandable and reflect reality, we can respond to them just as we would if they did not have dementia. By this phase of the condition, however, a person's speech may display some of the impairments described earlier. How should we respond to the person in these cases? We will consider two of the most common situations that may arise – unreal beliefs and confused speech.

Responding when the person expresses unreal beliefs

As stated earlier, memory impairment can be quite profound and the person may well find that their remaining memories are muddled, or they may mix up their memories of the past with the present. This can lead to their believing things to be true that are no longer the case. A very common belief is that a significant person from the past, such as a parent, is still alive. How should we respond when a person with moderate dementia says, 'My mother is coming to see me today'? There are three broad ways that we could reply.

1. Reality orientation: we could of course correct the person and tell them that no, their mother won't be coming because she died many years ago. Some would label this kind of response as 'reality orientation' and would say that it is appropriate that people with dementia are assisted to keep in touch with current reality as much as possible. This may be the case in some instances, but consider the effect on the person of being given this news. It will at the very

least upset them to learn that their mother is dead. It will remind them that they are themselves cognitively impaired when they realise that they have forgotten such a significant event. And if the news is given in a harsh or critical way, the person will feel demeaned and belittled.

Consider also that the person will quickly forget what has been said to them and later on may again say that their mother is coming to visit. If those around them correct them again, they will again experience the upset and ill-being that will result. Some have compared this situation to experiencing bereavement over and over.

2. White lies: we may feel that the upset that this kind of response would cause is cruel to the person and we may prefer not to try to orientate them to this kind of harsh reality. But if we are to forgo reality orientation, how should we respond instead? One alternative is to go along with what the person believes and in effect lie to the person: 'Oh that's good, I'm glad she's coming. You'll have a nice time with her won't you?'

We have already raised the question of the use of deception with people with dementia. We have said that some people in some situations may regard telling 'white lies' as being acceptable if they help resolve difficult situations, such as preventing a person from driving when they are not safe to do so. Is a white lie, in the form of collusion with the person's unreal belief, a helpful response in this case?

One difficulty with this kind of collusion is that, once entered into, it is hard for family members and friends to extract themselves from it. They would in effect have to maintain the fiction every time the person raises the topic of their mother. Then, if the person becomes impatient or distressed that their mother hasn't yet arrived, another white lie will be needed to try to resolve the situation: 'Oh she's rung up to say her train's been cancelled and she'll come tomorrow instead.' This may cause the person more distress and family members and friends are also left with bad feelings.

On the other hand, if the white lie is accepted by the person and makes them feel better, is it a bad thing? We have observed in Chapter 3 that white lies are often part of everyday relationships. Such interactions provide a quick and straightforward means of responding to some potentially awkward situations.

3. Validation: a third way that we could respond to a person's unreal belief has been termed 'validation'. If we make such a response, we do not agree or disagree with the person's belief but we attempt to engage with them at the level of the feelings that underlie that belief. An example of a validating response in this case would be, 'Your mother's a lovely person, isn't she? You've always been very fond of her.' Such a response allows the person to talk about their feelings regarding the person from the past while hopefully distracting them from their unreal belief in the present. In this way their well-being is maintained and family members and friends can interact with them in a positive way.

    There is no hard and fast rule about how to respond to unreal beliefs – any of these approaches may be appropriate in different situations. Having a range of communication skills appropriate for people with moderate dementia will help families and friends maintain close relationships with them.

Responding to confused speech

Another common communication difficulty that people with moderate dementia may experience is when they have something they want to say but cannot express their message properly so that their speech appears to others to be confused.

'One time Mum tried to tell me something but it had gone and she put her head down and started to cry and I remember taking hold of her hand and saying, "It's OK." She said that what she wanted to say was "there" then she described it as "disappearing". She still had that awareness – she was so upset about it. When she couldn't get the words out right you did a lot of saying, "Don't worry Mum it doesn't matter," but it clearly mattered to her.'

Let's consider an example:

Suppose that Bob is being visited by his daughter and baby grandson. He reaches out and takes the boy's hand and says with a smile on his face: 'There now, that'll be a good, er... whatsname isn't it, one day that'll be...whatsit...up here like...won't you be now...' How can we help Bob get his message across?

We could respond by asking Bob to say his message again and he might be able to make it clearer second time around. However, he may find it even harder to express himself again and may even forget what it was that he wanted to say, leading to possible distress and a breakdown of communication. An alternative strategy that Bob's daughter could employ is to try to find the basic sense within his message and in a variation of validation, respond to the feelings that Bob is trying to express. Clues to that feeling may come from interpreting what Bob says and also from the way he says it – does he appear happy, sad or angry when making his speech?

In this case we can assume from his smile that Bob is trying to say something happy or jocular. Holding his grandson's hand indicates that the message is about the boy. Clues as to the message can be found in what he has said: 'one day...up here...won't you be...' Bob may be trying to say something like, 'You'll be a big strapping lad one day, won't you?'

If Bob's daughter can pick such clues up, she can make a response that reflects the sense of what he is saying: 'He'll be a big boy soon, won't he, Dad?' In this way Bob's feelings are acknowledged even if the whole of what he wanted to say was not perfectly understood.

The case of Bob that we have considered here is an example of the communication technique of *reflection* (sometimes called 'mirroring'), which in this context means identifying the basic sense of a person's communication and reflecting that sense back to the person. The childcare expert Penelope Leach (1979, p.416) has observed that we use reflection naturally with babies and toddlers – when a youngster says delightedly, 'doggy!', we automatically respond, 'Yes, there's a dog isn't there?' As our children grow older, however, Leach comments that we often give up reflection as a way of interacting and rarely use it in adulthood. Reflection is, however, a very powerful communication technique and forms the basis of many approaches to counselling. Hearing the sense of what we have said gives us a good feeling because we can see that the person has listened enough to be able to repeat the message back to us. We have it on good authority that the British Queen Elizabeth uses reflection extensively when meeting her subjects as a way of demonstrating interest in those subjects' lives!

Research has shown that reflection can be a very useful communication technique when interacting with people with moderate dementia. Repeating back their messages gives them a sense of acknowledgement and validation. Reflection is often best done at a simple level, for example:

Bob: 'Grand – er – thing – day (pointing generally outside).'

Daughter: 'It's a lovely day outside, isn't it?'

*

Daughter: 'Are you enjoying your tea, Dad?'

Bob: 'Right tasty. It's ummmm…taste (smacking his lips)… yes.'

Daughter: 'It tastes nice does it? That's good.'

Some readers may be wondering why we are advocating a communication technique with people with dementia that we characteristically use with very young children. Isn't this demeaning the person? We were warned earlier by Tom Kitwood

(1997) that we should avoid infantilisation as an example of malignant social psychology. We would argue, however, that we are not treating people with dementia in a childlike way if we use techniques such as reflection; we are simply borrowing a communication technique from one setting and applying it to another. It is an example of a transferable skill that many of us will have acquired as parents, and which may help us interact better with people with moderate dementia.

GIVING A MESSAGE TO A PERSON WITH MODERATE DEMENTIA

Family members and friends will often want to give messages to the person they are supporting. They will want to tell them things, ask them things and sometimes give them instructions that will help them carry out tasks and activities. How can we ensure that our messages get through to the person? We will need to use principles of dementia empathy if we are to maximise our chances of the person understanding and responding appropriately to our messages. This means remembering that the person's difficulties will affect attention, memory and executive function, and trying to shape our messages in ways that will compensate for those difficulties.

Let us suppose that Ron, a friend of Bob's, has come to visit him. There are some basic principles that Ron can apply to make his conversation with Bob successful and agreeable to both of them.

- The setting for the conversation should be arranged to assist Bob to attend and concentrate. Lights should be bright but not glaring and there should be minimal extraneous noises or distractions – remember that people with dementia find it particularly hard to selectively attend if there are too many things happening around them.

- Ron must ensure that Bob has his attention. This means approaching Bob slowly from the front, to give Bob time to focus. If Bob is sitting down and does not appear to have noticed that Ron is there, Ron could crouch down in front of Bob's chair so that Bob can look down at him – research suggests that people with dementia find it easier to attend in those circumstances.

- Ron should not assume that Bob knows who he is, even if Bob appears to recognise him. As we've suggested earlier, people with dementia often retain superficial social skills and can employ them even if they don't have full understanding of a situation. It will be helpful to Bob if Ron introduces himself and the purpose of his visit: 'Hello Bob, it's Ron, we used to play bowls together. I've come to see you to have a chat and see how you're getting on.' This helps Bob attend to the conversation more effectively.

- Ron's voice should be clear but not too loud. He should keep the conversation simple and specific. He should use reflection to acknowledge Bob's contributions to the conversation. If Bob's responses to what he says contain unreal beliefs or 'confused' speech, Ron should try the validating responses discussed earlier.

ASKING A PERSON WITH DEMENTIA QUESTIONS

Some people suggest that one shouldn't ask a person with moderate dementia questions because they may have difficulty finding an appropriate answer and become distressed as a result. We would not go as far as this. Research indicates that people with moderate dementia certainly can answer questions and express their views on a range of topics. It is important that they are enabled as much as possible to make choices about aspects of their lives, and asking them questions is normally necessary for them to exercise choice.

At the same time, it is important to ask people with moderate dementia questions in a way that they can answer. As suggested earlier, it is very easy to overestimate a person's cognitive abilities. Anything other than the most straightforward question would indeed be too difficult for them. Asking them about aspects of their past lives is unlikely to gain more than a perfunctory response. Questions should be set in the here and now and framed in such a way that the person can use the information to hand in order to make a reply. Even a question such as 'What would you like to drink?' or 'Which dress would you like to wear today?' can be too hard for the person, because they may not remember the range of possible options. Framing such questions in the form, 'Would you like tea or coffee?' or 'Would you like to wear this dress or that dress?' (while showing the person the dresses) is a realistic way of enabling the person to make choices.

COMMUNICATION SKILLS FOR PROMOTING INDEPENDENCE AND ACTIVITY

People with moderate dementia can retain some independence in daily living skills such as washing, dressing, going to the toilet, and eating and drinking, but they may need some help and guidance to do so. Similarly, as we will discuss later, they can take part in activities but again may need assistance and direction. What communication skills do family members and friends need in order to assist people with moderate dementia to be independent and active? Broadly speaking, we will need to give them instructions and guidance. The following are some basic principles that may be useful:

- Begin by orientating the person to the task or activity, even if it is one they do several times a day: 'It's eight o'clock mother, I'm going to help you get dressed now.' It may be that the person will need to be reorientated at times during the activity.

- Remember that the person may not be able to comprehend abstract ideas, or even familiar things that are not in their field of view. Complement your verbal instructions by showing the person the dress you are going to help them put on, or the cup you are going to put their drink into. The person may not remember where the kitchen is and when taking them there it may be helpful to break down the journey into stages: 'We're going through the door here into the hall' (pointing towards the door); 'We're just turning into this room here' (pointing the way again).

- Breaking a task down into its constituent parts and slowly talking through the various stages will help overcome executive function issues. Keeping a flow of instructions will help the person attend and remain orientated.

- Sometimes a person will not at first understand or respond to even simple instructions. It is easy for family members or friends to get frustrated with them and even angry when this happens. It is important not to do so because the person will pick up on that frustration and may become more alarmed and agitated as a consequence. A good approach in this situation is to calmly repeat the instruction, perhaps wording it in a slightly different way. If the person still does not respond, wait a second or two and repeat it again. It may take a few goes, but they will usually pick up the message before too long.

As well as relationships, human activity is governed by communication and language and, by using simple principles such as these, families and friends can help people retain as much choice and independence as possible and carry out satisfying activities. We will move on to consider the range of social and leisure activities that a person with moderate dementia may be able to take part in, with the help of family members and friends.

Social and leisure activities for people with moderate dementia

In Chapter 3 we considered how to help people with early dementia remain active. We made the point that many people with early dementia can, with assistance, maintain some or all of the activities that they enjoyed prior to developing dementia. As the person moves towards the phase of moderate dementia, their increasing cognitive difficulties will affect their ability to engage in their accustomed activities.

> 'So after doing some artwork in daycare, he would come home and would tear up his painting and throw it in the bin. He had problems with this visual-spatial awareness; the upper left side was all blank, and so the painting was just all down the right side and along the bottom. He knew it was rubbish and he came home in a worse temper than when he went there.'

Some things will have to be given up and others will need to be adapted for a person with moderate dementia to be able to take part in them. It may also be that the person will respond better to activities that they have not recently been used to doing. The role of family members and friends (and professionals) becomes more important in helping the person remain active.

When teaching student nurses about activities for people with moderate dementia, we sometimes play a little game with them. We go round the room asking each student to think of one activity that such a person could do, with help. The catch is that they have to go through the alphabet, each student in turn coming up with an activity beginning with the next letter. Here's one list that was generated this way:

- Contact with **A**nimals
- Playing **B**owls
- Going to **C**hurch
- **D**ominoes
- **E**gg painting
- Watching an old **F**ilm
- **G**ardening
- Helping with **H**ousework
- Eating **I**ce-cream
- Making **J**elly

- **K**nitting
- Making things out of **L**ego
- Enjoying **M**usic
- **N**eedlework
- **O**rigami
- Going to the **P**ub
- **Q**uoits
- **R**eading
- **S**inging
- **T**rips out
- Washing **U**p (all right, that's a bit of a cheat!)
- Arranging flowers in a **V**ase (another cheat!)
- **W**alking
- Playing a **X**ylophone
- **Y**oga
- Visiting the **Z**oo

Try our game yourselves – the chances are you'll come up with a completely different list! The point is that the range of activities that can be done with people with moderate dementia is very wide. However, family members and friends will need imagination and skill in order to help them gain satisfaction and well-being from taking part in activities. We also need to be careful that activities are relevant for each particular person and sensitive to their changing abilities.

Consider our list of activities carefully. They represent a range of types of activity. Many can be done within the home (or in a residential care setting), while some involve going out. Some activities may be regarded as age specific – they are what older people who do not have dementia might take part in. Others do not seem so immediately appropriate for older people (such as making things out of LEGO®). Some could be done by a person on their own but many would need to involve other people. Several might also need to be simplified for a person with moderate dementia to be able to take part. Finally, some, such as housework or washing up are not really social or leisure based, but they are activities that a person may have been used to doing in the past and can still gain satisfaction from because they involve helping others. We will lump our long list of activities into broad groupings and consider each group in turn:

- Going out: activities that involve a person (with the assistance of others) going to places and doing things outside the place they live.

- Helping out: activities in which a person does things for others, or helps out around the house.

- Exercising: as the name suggests, activities that involve physical exercise.

- Activities of daily living: this grouping includes all aspects of a person meeting their own care needs, such as washing, dressing, eating and drinking.

- Sights and sounds: watching television, films or videos; listening to music or the radio.

- Pastimes: embracing hobbies, interests and games; pets and other animals.

GOING OUT

In Chapter 3 we encouraged family members and friends to assist a person with early dementia to go out and socialise. As the person moves towards moderate dementia, this may become more challenging. Their conversational skills will be impaired and other aspects of their social abilities may also be damaged, possibly leading to embarrassing situations. They may lack awareness of where they are or where they are going to, and they may need a lot of assistance to maintain safety. They may be experiencing difficulties using the toilet (see Chapter 5). Also, their memory and attention may be impaired to the point where they can only concentrate for a brief period of time. Given all these challenges, families, friends and professional carers may feel that taking a person with moderate dementia out of their usual living setting is 'too hard'.

It would be a shame, however, if this view prevailed. 'Trips out' are good for people with moderate dementia, as they are good for the rest of us, although family members and friends should remember two key principles when taking such a person out:

- Don't be too ambitious. Short, simple excursions are the most likely to be successful. The person's memory and attention difficulties may mean that they are unlikely to be able to appreciate long or intellectually complex outings and may tire easily. For example, a person may have enjoyed visiting museums or going to sports matches, but during the phase of moderate dementia outings may need to be adapted to shorter visits. A short walk, a visit to a public garden, a brief church service or a quick visit to a pub or café are more likely to be appreciated by the person, particularly if those with them help them to enjoy the excursion by engaging them in conversation and pointing out interesting aspects of their surroundings.

- Be prepared. Planning the trip beforehand will help to make it a success, as will taking with you things that the person may need, particularly regarding their continence needs. Anticipating any issues that their behaviour may cause others is also important (see Chapter 5), but families and friends should not be put off by the possibility of the person not always 'keeping up appearances', so long as others are not inconvenienced.

HELPING OUT

Many people with dementia will in the past have spent a lot of their time and gained satisfaction and well-being from doing things around the house, such as cooking, cleaning, gardening, DIY, or doing things for others. By the time they reach the phase of moderate dementia, they may have lost the ability to cook a meal or decorate a room or keep their garden in pristine condition. Some will also lose interest in such activities, but others will want to continue to help out and family members and friends should look for ways of assisting them to do so.

To achieve this, we must exercise dementia empathy skilfully and sensitively by finding things that the person can do that are within their capabilities. Trial and error may be involved here. People with moderate dementia engage better with activities that they can understand and respond to and this often means simple and straightforward things. For example, a person who likes cooking may be able to help cut up vegetables, or decorate an iced cake with sweets. Someone who enjoyed housework could assist with dusting or washing up and a keen gardener may enjoy deadheading flowers or watering plants. The person may need assistance and supervision even with such simple tasks, and families and friends should not expect perfect results – the activity is more important than the finished product.

> 'Dad gradually took over the cooking but he would sit Mum at the kitchen table and let her do things so she felt like she was taking a lead.'

> 'I think it's important that my husband still feels that he is part of our routine. For example, he always gets up before me and sets the table. He doesn't always get it right but I still let him do it.'

EXERCISING

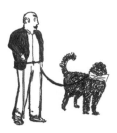

We have mentioned previously the importance of physical exercise for people with dementia. Exercise is good for a person's physical health; it may slow the progression of the condition and will reduce restlessness and sleep disturbances. If the person has been used to taking exercise, they are likely to want to continue to do so and, even if they have not valued exercise in the past, the benefits outlined earlier may encourage family members and friends to assist them with getting some exercise.

Walking is perhaps the best form of exercise for an older person with moderate dementia and we have mentioned it earlier. Even a short walk around the neighbourhood done regularly will be beneficial to the person. Some people with dementia appear to have a considerable need to walk around – we sometimes refer to this as 'wandering' and regard it as a problem, but it can be channelled in a positive way (so-called 'wandering' is discussed in Chapter 5). Other forms of exercise may be possible, such as visiting a swimming pool.

Within the home there are other opportunities for physical activity, taking into account both the person's cognitive and physical abilities. They may enjoy simple aerobic exercises or yoga, or spending time on an exercise bike. Ball games such as carpet bowls or simple games of catch will be within the person's capabilities and can be surprisingly enjoyable!

ACTIVITIES OF DAILY LIVING

A person with moderate dementia is likely to need assistance with daily living activities such as washing and bathing, dressing, eating and drinking. Those caring for the person, both family members and professional home or residential care staff, may regard providing such assistance as a chore or a task to be completed as quickly and efficiently as possible. Often this means doing for the person things that they could do for themselves, given enough time and appropriate help. It is our view that it is better if people with moderate dementia are allowed and assisted to meet as many as possible of their daily living needs themselves. Encouraging independence, as we have seen earlier, is very beneficial for people with dementia. It helps them retain skills and abilities for longer and may slow progression of the condition (psychologists refer to this as the 'use it or lose it' principle). Also, doing things for themselves leads to enhanced well-being. For many of us, activities of daily living are more than chores: they are enjoyable aspects of our lives. We like to choose what to wear and to get ourselves looking our best. We may enjoy relaxing in a bath and we look forward to meal times and drinks. People with dementia enjoy these things too.

To assist with this, the principles of dementia empathy should again be employed. Activities of daily living such as getting dressed make demands on the person's executive function abilities because they involve decision making and doing things in sequence. Those caring for a person with moderate dementia should take steps to simplify tasks for them. As we suggested earlier, such people can make choices so long as they are immediate ones, so asking the person, 'What dress do you want to wear?' may be too difficult. If, however, the person is shown two dresses and asked, 'Would you like to wear this one or that one?', or two different tops are laid out on view, then the person can exercise choice.

Executive function difficulties can lead to a person getting muddled when dressing themselves, so laying out clothes in the order that they need to put them on, or handing them items one after the other will help them dress themselves appropriately. Similar assistance could be provided with washing and doing hair, as well as make-up and jewellery, if the person wants to wear them.

'One morning my dad put a patterned skirt with a flowered blouse on Mum which didn't go; my mum would never have worn anything like that, and she went mad. She just looked at me and if she could have she'd have said, "Don't take me out looking like a fool." Dad didn't know what to do, so I sorted her wardrobe out into colour co-ordinations for him'.

The same principles of helping a person make realistic choices and assisting them to maintain independence can also be applied to mealtimes. These can of course also be opportunities for conversation and socialising. By the way, we are not averse to people with dementia drinking alcohol if that is what they have been used to – within recommended limits of course! We will discuss eating and drinking further in Chapter 5.

Another principle we have mentioned that applies to activities of daily living is to make allowances for a person not getting everything right and not to blame them if they make mistakes with dressing or have imperfect table manners. Our approach should be to tactfully help them along the right path.

SIGHTS AND SOUNDS

Television

Many people with dementia will of course have enjoyed watching television throughout their lives. For some, television would have been their main form of relaxation. To what extent can television watching continue to be an enjoyable pastime for people with moderate dementia?

For those caring for a person with dementia, whether in their home or in residential care, the temptation to sit the person in front of the television and expect them to watch it while the carer gets on with things is considerable. However, dementia empathy should tell us that television (and speech programmes on the radio) place considerable cognitive demands on the person and many programmes may be beyond their abilities. TV programmes demand memory, to follow plots and recognise characters. They are usually verbal in nature, placing demands on language skills.

Images change rapidly, making it hard for the person to keep up. It is not uncommon for people to misinterpret the images as being real, which may cause distress. TV programmes are also long when compared to the attention span of a person with moderate dementia. Small wonder that before too long the person has either fallen asleep or got up and walked off when left to watch TV.

Television viewing can however be an enjoyable activity for people with moderate dementia, if those caring for a person use it creatively. First, the development of video technology has led to the possibility of creating 'bespoke' programmes for people. Videos could be made of a person's family or friends, places that they know and like, or activities that they particularly enjoy. If such films are clear, simple and short, the person may gain great enjoyment from watching them. One such video can of course be shown to the person many times and it is best if family members or friends can sit with them and help them enjoy the video more by talking with them about the people and scenes as they appear in the 'programme'.

Another aspect of television watching is that family members and friends may be surprised by the kind of programme that a person may enjoy. The late Oxford University Professor of Philosophy and novelist Iris Murdoch developed dementia in her early 70s and was cared for by her husband John Bayley, himself a Professor at Oxford. In his book *Iris* (which was later made into a film), Bayley (1998, p.158) describes sitting on the sofa with Iris watching *Teletubbies*, a television programme that was aimed at an audience of toddlers. Iris, during the phase of moderate dementia, enjoyed *Teletubbies* and other children's programmes such as cartoons and, as Bayley put it, watched them with 'something approaching glee'.

We may be baffled and even disturbed by the image of two retired Oxford University professors sitting together watching programmes made for very young children. We may feel that it was wrong for Iris Murdoch's husband to encourage her to watch such programmes and that he was demeaning and infantalising her. Family members and friends may be appalled by the idea of the person they know and care for doing likewise.

We would urge those who hold such views to think again and use dementia empathy to see things from the point of view of the person with dementia. We have seen earlier that 'adult' television programmes are likely to be too complicated for people with moderate dementia to follow. Children's programmes, however, especially those for the youngest audience, are produced to a different set of assumptions. Programmes such as *Teletubbies* are simple, repetitive, contain few words and importantly are made up of bright, clear, colourful and straightforward images. People with moderate dementia may be attracted to such programmes because they are easy for them to understand and relate to. Enjoyment of such programmes does not mean that the person is 'going back to childhood'. Like the rest of us, they are simply gaining stimulation and enjoyment from watching and listening to something they can follow.

We are not suggesting that all people with moderate dementia should watch children's programmes. Everyone is of course different and some will relate to particular programmes more than others. We would suggest, however, that family members and friends think more flexibly about what a person may appreciate and enjoy and not dismiss programmes or activities aimed at young children. At the end of the day, the proof of the pudding is in the eating and we would commend John Bayley for having the vision and open-mindedness to realise how far through dementia Iris Murdoch had travelled and to enhance her well-being in this way. More commendable still is that he took the trouble to sit with her and made watching the programme a shared occasion. We will say more about the place of children's toys and games in dementia care later in this chapter.

Music

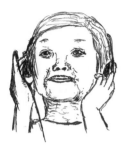

Music is of course an important aspect of many people's lives and again people with dementia are no exception. Research has shown the extent to which music can enhance the well-being of such people. Music may also help reduce incidences of behaviour that others find difficult by relaxing a person and giving them something agreeable to attend to. It has often been noted that people with moderate dementia may be able to sing along to the lyrics of songs that they know well, even when in other respects their memory and language difficulties are quite marked – no one really knows why this should be.

There are many ways that family members and friends may help a person with moderate dementia enjoy music. Playing music during the day that the person likes is of course the most straightforward means of achieving this aim, though as with most of us the music will soon seem to fade into the background and the person will stop attending to it. At the same time, relaxing background music can engender a good mood in a person.

Family members and friends may wish to make a shared activity out of music by sitting with a person and listening to particular pieces with them. Perhaps the person could be encouraged to sing along. If the person played a musical instrument, they could be assisted to continue to play, though they may well not have the facility that they used to. Some people like playing simple percussion instruments such as drums and tambourines (we mentioned xylophones earlier as part of our alphabetical list!). As with television programmes, we may sometimes find that the person relates better to less sophisticated music than they used to – we find that what we call 'sing-along' music often goes down well. By this we mean songs that the person may have sung at school or in organisations such as churches or community groups.

In order to encourage engagement and response, music is more likely to be of benefit if it is relevant to a person's preferences. We all no doubt have favourite pieces of music or songs that make us feel happy or sad but which are important to how we feel. However, approaches such as 'music therapy', which use classical or orchestral pieces, are also being increasingly recognised as beneficial. For people living with dementia, the use of music does seem to have a particularly significant role in supporting well-being and as such can be a very important activity, especially as a person's abilities diminish.

At the same time, we must recognise that the old are, as it were, getting younger – it won't be long before a generation of older people will come along that was brought up on music such as Heavy Metal or Punk Rock – posing new challenges for those caring for them!

PASTIMES

Perhaps all other activities that don't fit into one of the stated categories may be grouped together under the heading of 'pastimes'. This heading embraces all the hobbies, games and interests that a person enjoyed before they developed dementia. It may also include activities that are more often associated with childhood, such as dolls and toys. All the benefits of activity can be applied to the category of pastimes and families and friends can again enhance the well-being of the person by assisting them to enjoy such interests and games.

At the same time, we must again remember the principles of dementia empathy. Many pastimes that a person enjoyed in the past will be beyond their capabilities if they have moderate dementia. As we have suggested, card games, crosswords, quizzes, hobbies that involve making things or sports with complex rules may become difficult and will at least need to be adapted. For example, a person who enjoyed bowls may lose the ability to understand a match and the tactics involved. However, they may still be able to deliver a bowl accurately and so a simplified game could be played where the aim is just to get a single bowl nearest to the 'jack'. In the same vein, simpler games could be substituted for more complex ones – a person who previously enjoyed bridge may still be able to play snap. We have mentioned previously how people with dementia may be assisted to help out with such activities as gardening and cooking by being helped to carry out simple components of those activities, and the same may be applied to pastimes. For example, a person who previously knitted sweaters may be able to knit simple squares and a keen painter could still use colours and make patterns. As ever, family members and friends need to be flexible, creative and non-blaming – the pastime is more important than its outcome or product. As mentioned before though, sensitivity is required to make sure that the person does not become frustrated by not being able to carry out an activity with the same skill they used to. And of course we should not make the person carry out an activity they do not enjoy.

> 'When the Bingo apparatus came out at the day centre, my husband would make for the door at 100 miles an hour and the person in charge would say to me, like a head teacher to a parent, "He has been a bit difficult today." If I knew then what I know now, I would say, "Are you surprised, given the sort of activity you make him do?"'

Another aspect of pastime that people with dementia often enjoy is access to pets and other animals. Many will of course have been used to having pets and those caring for them may be able to help them continue to look after and gain pleasure from dogs, cats and other animals. If keeping a pet is not possible, family members and friends can enhance a person's well-being by bringing their own pets to visit them. As well as animals, many people with dementia enjoy the company of children and babies and family members and friends should not be afraid of bringing their children to visit them, though often short well-supervised visits may be better for the person and for the child.

We have discussed previously ways that a person's accustomed pastimes may be adapted to take account of moderate dementia and allow them to continue to enjoy those activities. There is a further aspect of pastime that may be appropriate. This is the use of dolls, toys or children's games as ways of promoting activity with people with dementia. This is an area that is clearly controversial, but research (some carried out by one of us) indicates that people with moderate dementia may derive considerable well-being from dolls or children's toys.

Dolls, particularly life-like ones, are often much appreciated by people with dementia. Some will 'adopt' a doll as if it were their own child and will take it around with them and look after it. Is this a good thing? Our view is that we see nothing wrong in a person with moderate dementia deriving well-being in this way. It will do the person no harm and 'looking after' a doll has the particular benefit of helping the person feel useful to another – something that in the 'real world' is denied them because of their own dependence on others. Lifelike toy dogs and cats can also enhance well-being in the same way.

Some professional or family carers have gone further and used a wide range of children's toys as means of promoting activity with people with moderate dementia. Particularly useful is the range of electronic dolls and toys that are now available. Examples from our own experience that have been enjoyed by people with dementia include a large furry toy duck that quacked 'Old MacDonald had a farm' when its wing was pressed, a toy parrot that repeated what someone said to it and a motorised toy dog that walked across the floor and yapped. In all cases, people with moderate dementia showed obvious enjoyment when 'playing' with these toys. For men, 'boys' toys' such as motorised cars and trains have also gone down well (recall that making things with LEGO was another of our alphabetical list of activities!). Still more enjoyment has been gained from such things as balloons and bubbles and even kazoos and party blowers.

What do we make of the use of children's toys and games with people with dementia? The issues are of course the same as those in the example we gave earlier of Iris Murdoch watching *Teletubbies*. Dolls and children's toys are bright, simple and understandable to people with moderate dementia. We ourselves have been surprised by the enthusiasm with which many people with dementia embrace dolls and toys and have had to modify our own feelings of discomfort when using them – again the proof of the pudding is in the eating and whatever promotes enjoyment and well-being can't be bad.

Summary: principles of promoting activity with people with moderate dementia

- Anything a person with dementia does is an activity: as we have seen, our definition of activity is a broad one, embracing daily living activities as well as pastimes and 'passive' activities such as watching television. The trick is to make whatever the person does an opportunity to promote engagement with others and enhance well-being.

- Make time for activities: it is easy to regard activities as an 'optional extra', to be done only if possible. Our view is that activities are integral to the well-being of a person and research has shown that the behaviour of people with dementia who are encouraged to be active causes fewer difficulties to others.

- Be prepared to participate: people with moderate dementia are rarely able to initiate activities and are likely to need assistance in carrying them out. Family members and friends should be prepared to participate in activities with a person and are likely to have to take the lead with many activities.

- Base activities on what a person has always liked to do: familiar activities are most likely to be enjoyed and the person may be better able to carry out activities they have been used to doing.

- Use dementia empathy to make activities achievable: activities need to be adapted, simplified and often shortened for people with moderate dementia.

- Make activities social occasions: take part in the activity yourself and encourage others to spend time with the person as well. Use activity times as opportunities for interaction and conversation.

- Encourage independence and choices: let a person choose activities or aspects of activity as much as possible and allow them to do as much for themselves as they can.

- Remember that the activity itself is more important than the outcome: it is not important if the painting that the person produces or the cake they ice is not perfect. It is the fact that the person is experiencing well-being through being active that is key.

- Consider dolls and toys: the value of dolls, toys and children's games for promoting well-being in people with moderate dementia is well established by research and the experience of many carers. If we can move beyond our reservations, we may find that a person will benefit from such things to a much greater extent than we think they will.

- Ask for help and involve others: for family carers who are doing a lot of the caring, it is important to ask others for help and support with activities because it is an ideal way in which others can get involved and provide a valuable break. Equally, for those who are less involved, it is really helpful to suggest an activity you can do with the person, because the main carer may find it difficult to ask for help.

CHAPTER 5

The Challenges of Moderate Dementia

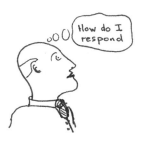

There are a number of challenges that people living with moderate dementia and their families and friends might have to face. These can be caused by physical changes as a result of dementia or changes in comprehension, behaviour and ways of coping. Some changes can be particularly challenging and upsetting for family and friends who are supporting a person and we will address these under the broad heading of behaviours that others find difficult. In addition, specific attention will be given to the challenges of eating and drinking, using the toilet and the potential difficulties of admission into hospital when someone has moderate dementia. Finally, we will consider the sensitive issues of vulnerability and abuse.

Behaviour that others find difficult

We have chosen the heading for this section with care. We wish to avoid terms sometimes found in books for families or professional carers such as 'behaviour problems' or 'challenging behaviour'.

Such terms seem to imply that the difficulty is with the person with dementia; that they are somehow doing something wrong and their behaviour should be clamped down upon. We might even, when using such terms, come to feel that the person is in some way to blame for their behaviour. This is rarely the case with people with moderate dementia. When family members and friends feel challenged by the person's manner or actions, it is important for them to remember that the person may intend something very different by those actions from how it comes across to others. In other words, it isn't that the person is being 'difficult' – they are simply trying to relate to their world. At the same time, there is no doubt that *others* may find the person's behaviour difficult and may experience considerable feelings of stress as a result. Coping with such behaviour is a major issue for family members and friends of people with moderate dementia, for this is the phase of dementia when it is most likely to occur. However, significant caution should be observed if there is a sudden increase in such things as agitated or distressed behaviour. Such changes may be the result of a physical health issue such as an infection, constipation or dehydration, or a change in the person's medication. This may lead to their experiencing *delirium* (see Chapter 2) and this should be ruled out and treated if found to be the cause.

WHAT DO FAMILIES AND FRIENDS FIND DIFFICULT?

Broadly speaking, we can identify five main categories of behaviour that families and friends may find difficult. These categories overlap somewhat and a person's behaviour may sometimes fall into several of them:

- When the person lacks awareness that their actions will put them at risk of coming to harm.

- When the person's manner and actions indicate that they are in distress.

- When the person behaves in ways that are considered socially inappropriate.

- When the person tries to get their needs met through behaving aggressively or with hostility.

- When the person seems to be unwilling to accept help from others and their basic needs such as eating and drinking or using the toilet are compromised.

We will explore these categories in more detail below. Before we do so, however, we will consider a more fundamental question.

WHAT CAUSES PEOPLE WITH MODERATE DEMENTIA TO BEHAVE IN WAYS THAT OTHERS FIND DIFFICULT?

We can offer two possible broad explanations that may underlie such changes in behaviour:

- The person's behaviour is a symptom of dementia.

- The person is trying to get their needs met.

The person's behaviour is a symptom of dementia

It used to be thought that more or less all 'problem behaviour' was essentially a symptom of dementia. This implied that such behaviour was random and meaningless and simply a result of damage to the brain. If the person had a strong urge to walk about, it was known as 'wandering'; it was felt that there was no purpose behind the activity and the person was not heading for any destination. If a person acted in an aggressive way, it was again thought that these were essentially random outbursts that neither they nor others could control.

It is true that in most cases a person would not behave in these ways if they did not have dementia and family members and friends are often acutely aware of the extent that the person's manner and actions have changed since its onset. It is also the case that some actions are hard for others to understand or interpret. Also, as we saw in Chapter 2, some types of dementia such as fronto-temporal dementia affect areas of the brain particularly associated with manner and behaviour, leading to increased likelihood of the person behaving in socially inappropriate or puzzling ways, which can cause upset.

It can also be tempting for family members and friends, when faced with behaviour that is causing difficulties, to believe that the person is acting deliberately and to blame them for their manner. 'He's always been an awkward so-and-so and he still is' was how one exasperated relative put it. Again, there is a grain of truth in this perspective. Many of us may be regarded by others as 'awkward so-and-so's' from time to time and relationships between those who do not have dementia do not of course always run smoothly. Not all people with dementia experience changes in manner and some who have had issues with relationships in the past may appear to continue to do so. However, we must again be careful before apportioning blame to the person. As we have seen, awareness or comprehension will be impaired for most people with moderate dementia and similarly awareness of the consequences of behaviour may not be recognised.

The person is trying to get their needs met

Research is increasingly showing that much of the behaviour that others find difficult is not random and meaningless and is not a deliberate attempt to be awkward. It is simply that the person has some inner need that, because of their condition, they cannot express or meet in a conventional way. Sometimes the need is an immediate one; for example, a person may become concerned and agitated because they need the toilet or are in pain. Sometimes the need reflects aspects of the person's life history, such as a person who lived on a farm expressing a need to be outdoors. Family members and friends can often use their knowledge of the person, along with principles of dementia empathy, to identify the need underlying the person's behaviour and use that understanding to help them get their needs met. Our view is that when faced with behaviour that they find difficult, families and friends should always assume in the first instance that the person's manner and actions are meaningful in this way, rather than that the person's behaviour is random, or just a symptom of their dementia. Only if it is clear that no meaning can be found in the person's behaviour should other explanations be sought.

> 'My husband used to shake his fist and swear at himself in the mirror. Years later I understood what was going on. He couldn't recognise himself because, with recent memories erased, he thought he was a young man again, and also, because of visual-spatial problems, he thought the reflection was a real person. He was thinking: "Who is this stranger in my house?" Maybe he thought, "My wife is being unfaithful."'

When the person lacks awareness that their actions will put them at risk of coming to harm

We discussed in Chapter 3 how a person with early dementia may, by trying to carry on with their accustomed lives, put themselves at risk of harm. A person living alone may forget to turn the gas off after making a meal; a person who tries to drive when their judgement is impaired may risk having an accident, and so on. By the phase of moderate dementia, such risks may have diminished because the person's declining abilities and awareness mean that such independent actions are less likely to occur. However, that decline in abilities and awareness carries its own risks as the person becomes more and more reliant on others. One aspect of risk is that of abuse or exploitation by others, which we will consider later. But the 'risky behaviour' that family members and friends are often most concerned about is when the person has a profound need to be on their feet and to walk about, but lacks awareness of where they are or how to get from one place to another – and, more importantly, how to get back safely. As we have seen, such walking about is often called 'wandering'.

We dislike this term because it implies aimlessness, whereas, as we discussed earlier, the person is likely to be fulfilling an inner need by walking about. That need may be related to their current situation: perhaps they are experiencing pain or discomfort. Often walking about derives from boredom, if the person's day is empty. Sometimes they simply want some exercise. If the period of walking is prolonged, it could be that they have forgotten how long they have been on their feet.

Other explanations for walking about may derive from a person's life history. We mentioned previously a farmer who had always been used to being outside. The person may have had a job that involved being on their feet, or recreational walking may have always been an important part of their life.

The chief risk associated with walking about is of course the possibility of the person getting lost. An associated risk is that they may fall, especially if they are becoming physically frail. If they want to go outdoors, they may become frustrated if they cannot do so and act aggressively as a consequence, thereby compounding the difficulty experienced by those caring for them.

How should we respond when a person displays such behaviour? As they have a clear need to walk about, our response should be to find ways of their doing so safely rather than preventing them from being active. Ideally, family members and friends will find time to take them out for walks – as we saw earlier, exercise is good for all people with dementia. If a person's main carer is less physically active, then other family members or friends could perhaps go out with them. Providing activities during the day and involving the person in what is going on may reduce boredom. If they were previously less active, investigations for pain or other possible physical causes of restlessness should be carried out. Steps could be taken to allow them to walk about indoors safely by clearing ways and removing obstacles that they could fall over.

What if a person is insistent on going outside when it is not possible for someone to go with them? Increasingly assistive technology is playing a role in keeping people safe while allowing them freedom to walk outside by making available devices that individuals carry on their person. These devices, similar to mobile phones in appearance, act as a tracking system that allows others to find out where the person is. Alternatively, a simpler option may be to have a label or necklace, which provides emergency information should they get lost.

For those who are considered unsafe to go out alone, some carers would resort to locking the door (making sure it could be opened quickly in an emergency, such as a fire). This may be sufficient to put some people off, but others may become more upset and frustrated as they try in vain to open the door and more creative approaches may need to be tried. Perhaps it is possible for a person to go into the garden on their own, if the gate to the road is locked. Sometimes it is possible to disguise a door so that a person does not realise where it is. These are drastic measures, but those caring for people with dementia may perhaps be excused for putting safety first.

When the person's manner and actions indicate that they are in distress

People with moderate dementia can experience the full range of emotions but sometimes, because of their intellectual and language difficulties, they are not able to clearly express how they are feeling. Their emotions may, however, be reflected in their behaviour. It is always worth considering if a person might be in pain or physically unwell yet unable to express this. It is not uncommon for older people in particular to have other conditions that cause them discomfort such as arthritis, gastric problems or dental pain. If a person is distressed, it is important to establish if there is a physical cause so that this can be treated. If this proves difficult though, offering mild pain relief and observing its effect is often worth a try.

We have seen earlier that walking about may be a sign of boredom. It could also be that the person is feeling anxious, perhaps half remembering events from the past and believing that they should be doing something. Anxiety is a not uncommon feeling among people with moderate dementia. As their awareness declines, the world can become a confusing and even frightening place as they become increasingly unable to understand what is happening to them and what is going on around them. Anxiety may manifest itself in the person becoming restless and agitated, asking questions over and over, and continually seeking the presence and reassurance of familiar people. Family members and friends may understandably find such behaviour tiring and frustrating.

> 'My husband became quite anxious, partly because I became crosser with him. I would say: "You have just asked me that – you've asked me that eight times today." I am not a very patient person.'

Restlessness may also result from the environment that the person is living in. We have discussed previously that a person's attention difficulties will make noisy and overactive environments stressful. If they do not understand where they are or how to find places such as the toilet, their anxiety may again be increased.

Anxiety may also be a consequence of a person experiencing symptoms such as hallucinations or delusions or misinterpreting their environment. As we discussed in Chapter 1, hallucinations are false perceptions, in which a person sees things that are not there, or hears voices apparently saying things to them. Delusions are false beliefs: a person firmly believing something to be true that is not actually the case. Equally they may have disturbances to their visual perception, which makes them misinterpret what they are seeing. All these things may cause a person distress if the perception or belief is unpleasant, sad or frightening.

It is important that those caring for a person use dementia empathy to try to appreciate why they are feeling the way they do. Difficult though it can sometimes be, one should also try to remain calm and reassuring, as if we show our anger or frustration it will almost certainly increase the person's anxiety. Spending quality time with them, including them in what is going on and keeping them orientated by telling them what is happening on a regular basis may help to reassure and calm them.

Another emotion that people with moderate dementia may experience is depression. Research indicates that depression is at its most common during this phase and anything up to 25 per cent of people with dementia may experience depression at some time. A person may not be able to express their feelings verbally but depression may result in their becoming upset and tearful, or may lead to their appearing to be withdrawn, unmotivated or apathetic. Alternatively they may become more agitated and restless. The best way that families and friends can help is by giving them time and love and encouraging them to do some activities – psychologists tell us that trying to stay active is one of the best medicines for those who are depressed. Anti-depressant drugs may be considered useful if a person's depression is very profound and/or other approaches have been exhausted.

When the person behaves in ways that are socially inappropriate

Family members and friends can become very upset if a person's manner and actions are not socially appropriate – when they are rude, messy, untidy, over-talkative or disinhibited, or alternatively when they appear to be lacking in interest in things. Dementia empathy should again assure us that the person cannot help the way they are: such behaviour is a manifestation of loss of cognitive abilities. In particular, executive function impairment will affect a person's judgement in social situations. Up to a point, the best strategy is to make allowances for them – as someone once put it, on no account try to keep up appearances. Sometimes those caring for the person create problems for themselves by expecting too much of them or by insisting that things should be as they were before the person developed dementia – understandable though it is that families should wish that this was so.

At the same time, we are not suggesting that socially inappropriate behaviour should be totally ignored. For one thing, people with dementia do not want to be the way they are. If they could magically be cured of dementia and look back at the way they had been behaving, they may be shocked, embarrassed and upset. Family members and friends sometimes need to uphold a person's dignity by gently correcting or diverting them if they start to act in ways that upset others, or would upset themselves if they knew what they were doing.

'I think a couple of our neighbours have found it quite difficult. My husband sometimes says things that are inappropriate due to the nature of his dementia and he must have said something rude to a neighbour. One day he (the neighbour) avoided us both in the street; he had previously ignored my husband but not me. So I wrote to him explaining the reason.'

This particularly applies when, as sometimes happens, a person becomes sexually disinhibited and starts making inappropriate advances towards someone else (discussed in Chapter 3). In all cases it is important to maintain respect for the person and not to abandon them if they do not always act the way they used to.

Loss of interest in activities may reflect the fact that a person is depressed or that the suggested activity is now too hard for them to understand and appreciate. Attempting to find briefer and simpler activities may be appropriate, and we may have to accept that the person's world is shrinking.

'I think the thing we found hardest wasn't Grandma forgetting things but the lack of interest she has in life, the things she used to enjoy like going to garden centres: if you take her now she'll just walk behind you, she won't look around her and see what's there… The majority of the time Grandma will just sit there and gaze into space but I don't think she has the same awareness of time, she gets lost in her own head thinking about things and I don't think it's as horrendous as others think.'

When the person tries to get their needs met by behaving aggressively or with hostility

Unsurprisingly, this is an aspect of dementia that causes particular stress for carers. Aggressive behaviour includes verbal threats, swearing and hostile utterances, and physical aggression, such as hitting, slapping, spitting and scratching. It is fortunately rare that a person with dementia seriously injures another, but it can happen, particularly if they are being cared for by someone who is themselves an older person. Those with young-onset dementia can be particularly prone to responding to events in an aggressive way and, being younger, they can potentially cause more injury by doing so.

Sadly, aggression is a fact of everyday life. How often have we found ourselves being shouted at in a family row, been on the receiving end of an angry driver's blaring horn or had to manage an irate customer at work? How often have we been the ones dishing out the aggression in these situations? Most of us have the potential to act aggressively if we are threatened, frustrated or our needs are not being met. People with dementia are no different from the rest of us, but because of their condition they may act aggressively in a wider range of situations than they would have done, as a result of their cognitive and language difficulties preventing them from getting their needs met in more appropriate ways.

People with dementia are rarely aggressive for no reason. Usually, aggressive behaviour happens in response to an outside event that acts as a *trigger*. Sometimes, family members and friends can themselves trigger aggression if they approach the person in an angry or blaming way. It may be that relationships within the family have always been volatile with frequent arguments and, if these continue when the person develops dementia, then actual physical aggression may result. Interacting with a potentially aggressive person requires a calm and reassuring manner. The qualities of patience and acceptance are never more important than when the person is prone to acting aggressively.

> 'Suddenly it was much easier; I had been trying to take over but I suddenly realised that some of my husband's aggression was because I was being too bossy – "Come on, put your shoes on" – treating him like a child.'

Aggression may result if a person is being helped to do something they don't want to do, or don't understand the reason for. A common trigger for aggression is when others are trying to give personal care, such as helping the person wash or dress (see later). Conversely, aggressive behaviour may arise if the person is being prevented from doing something that they wish to do, such as going outside when it is not convenient for them to do so.

Aggression can result from the person not understanding their situation and feeling frightened and vulnerable. Understanding the underlying need that they are expressing is the first step to making an appropriate response.

When the person seems to be unwilling to accept help from others

People with moderate dementia often need considerable assistance with daily living activities, but may not always be willing to accept such assistance. As we have seen, they may resist when being helped to get washed and dressed or when those caring for them want them to go somewhere, and they may respond aggressively if pressed. This not unnaturally causes frustration in carers.

If such situations arise, we should again try to understand the situation from the person's perspective, to see if we can identify reasons for their resistance. It may be that they were approached in the wrong way, or not given enough orientation to what the carer was intending to do and felt threatened and defensive as a result. Perhaps they did not recognise who was with them, even though it was someone very familiar to them, or perhaps they just didn't want to get dressed at that moment, thank you very much!

Those caring for a person can try a range of approaches when the person is resistive in this way. First and foremost, is it possible to respect their wishes not to be disturbed – do they have to get washed or dressed at that time?

'My husband went through a phase of not wanting to take off his jogging bottoms, and went to bed in them. So we had these scenes with me saying, "Come on, you have to take your trousers off before going to bed," but the outreach worker said: "There is no law against going to bed in your tracksuit bottoms," so suddenly that problem disappeared, because someone told me how to deal with it – it was my problem, not his – just let it go.'

Sometimes leaving a person and coming back later is all that is required. If the activity of daily living is necessary, trying to orientate the person as much as possible may help. This could involve a clear explanation of what is wanted, perhaps reinforced by visual cues – for example, holding the dress up so they can see it. As discussed previously, involving the person in the activity and offering choices and opportunities for them to do things for themselves may enhance co-operation. If they do not appear to understand instructions, repeating those instructions calmly and clearly, perhaps changing the wording a little, may help the message get through.

> 'My husband was also "whopping me one" so when the carer was washing him I was holding his hands and singing to him, talking to him and distracting him while the carer was getting on with the job. Then another carer came once a week to give him a bath. He disliked showers because he thought it was somebody hitting him so he hit back.'

The role of medication

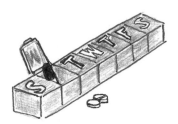

Despite the range of interpersonal approaches available to family members and friends for smoothing relationships with people with moderate dementia, a person may still act in ways that cause difficulties, frustration and stress for those caring for them. In these circumstances desperate carers often see medication as being the answer and will appeal to their doctor to give the person 'something to calm them down'. GPs will frequently be at a loss to suggest alternatives and will often acquiesce to such requests.

Three broad types of medication are available that may make a person's manner and behaviour less difficult for others. First, there is some evidence that the ACEI drugs given to people in the early to moderate phases of dementia (see Chapter 2) may help by making them better orientated to their surroundings and therefore less prone to being resistant or defensive due to misunderstanding. Another drug called memantine (Namenda or Ebixa) is available for people with moderate to advanced dementia and is aimed at reducing occurrences of 'difficult behaviour'. Current evidence is that the effects of all these drugs are modest. Recent research has suggested that over-the-counter pain killers given on a regular basis may be just as effective in modifying behaviour, suggesting that much agitation and aggression may be the result of the person experiencing pain or physical discomfort (though medical advice should be sought before these are given, because of potential side effects).

Second, anxiolytic drugs may sometimes be prescribed in an attempt to treat anxiety, in particular drugs from the benzodiazepine group such as diazepam (Valium) or lorazepam (Ativan). These may help in the short term, but in most cases anxiety is a long-term feeling for people with dementia and these drugs are ineffective and potentially harmful if given for more than a few weeks. There is also particular concern about the prescription of these drugs to frail older people because of the increased risk of unsteadiness and falls.

The third broad group of drugs often prescribed for people with dementia are so-called 'anti-psychotic' drugs. Examples include risperidone, olanzapine and quetiapine. These are most commonly prescribed for people with severe mental illnesses such as schizophrenia and bipolar disorder. However, they are sometimes used with people with dementia because they have sedative properties and are supposed to make a person less agitated and restless and thereby less prone to aggression. They are also intended to reduce the occurrence of hallucinations and delusions.

The prescription of anti-psychotic drugs to people with dementia is becoming increasingly controversial and there are calls to minimise the use of such drugs as a human rights issue. While they may quieten agitated people to an extent, they have many unwanted effects. They can increase a person's sense of confusion, making it harder for those caring for the person to interact meaningfully with them. According to a recent UK review by the Alzheimer's Society (2011), anti-psychotic drugs increase the risk of many harmful physical conditions or events, including Parkinsonism, falls, dehydration, chest infections, ankle oedema, deep vein thrombosis/pulmonary embolism, cardiac arrhythmia and stroke. It has become established that people with dementia who take anti-psychotic drugs have higher death rates, largely due to increased incidence of pneumonia and life-threatening blood clots related to sedation.

In short, anti-psychotic drugs offer few benefits in terms of minimising behaviour that causes difficulty to others and can sometimes have life-threatening side effects. Current guidelines in the UK and other English-speaking countries are that such drugs should only be prescribed when a person's behaviour is causing extreme distress to themselves or others and all other avenues have been explored; and in fact only one drug, risperidone, is now licensed for this use in the UK. In the USA, the Food and Drug Administration has stated that anti-psychotic drugs are not approved for dementia-related symptoms. Prescriptions should be reviewed every few weeks and no great expectations should be held that the drugs will do anything other than sedate the person.

> 'When my husband shouted and swore at his reflection he was given haloperidol [an anti-psychotic]; it increased his confusion and caused him to shuffle, and it brought on a mild heart attack, when all I should have done was take the mirrors down. Again it was everyone's ignorance about what can trigger aggressive behaviour.'

Hard-pressed families and friends are unlikely to be pleased to read this conclusion. While the interpersonal strategies discussed in this section (and summarised below) can help relations with a person with moderate dementia considerably, there is no doubt that family members and friends can remain troubled by aspects of the person's behaviour and those caring for them can experience considerable stress and burden as a result of their manner and actions. Research has shown that these issues are the main reasons why informal caring relationships break down and residential care is sought for the people concerned.

This implies that, if given appropriately, anti-psychotic medication may on occasion be a necessary and helpful option in providing a way to reduce distressing symptoms and avoid breakdown in the caring situation. As one man who has dementia recently said to one of us:

> 'I was being aggressive towards my wife and, if it hadn't been for the fact I was given an anti-psychotic which calmed me down, my wife would have never have spoken to me again *or* continued supporting me. That would have been much worse than the risks of taking it!'

Summary: how should family members and friends respond when they find a person's manner and actions difficult?

- Remember that the person almost certainly does not mean to be difficult. They are trying to fulfil a need that they cannot express in a conventional way.

- Adopt a calm and reassuring approach. Don't argue with the person or raise your voice, even when you are feeling frustrated by their behaviour. Don't be the trigger that causes an aggressive outburst.

- Ensure that the environment is calming and orientating.

- Use dementia empathy to try to ascertain the meaning behind the person's actions. What need are they trying to fulfil and does it relate to their present circumstances or to their past life?

- Check that the person's behaviour is not due to pain or physical discomfort.

- Reduce the person's anxiety by including them in events. Try to keep them orientated to their surroundings and what is happening around them.

- Be flexible and tolerant. Find ways of allowing the person to walk about safely. Don't insist on their doing things they are refusing to do, unless it is absolutely necessary.

- Involve the person in regular activities and exercise. It will relieve boredom, use up excess energy and may lift their mood.

- Ask for medication only as a last resort and don't expect too much from it. Look out for signs that the person is experiencing side effects of medication.

Challenges to eating and drinking

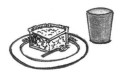

We all need to eat and drink and nearly all of us enjoy eating and drinking. People with dementia are of course no different, but by the phase of moderate dementia a person is likely to need assistance meeting their nutritional needs. In this section we will consider how those caring for the person can help them eat a good diet and gain satisfaction from food and drink.

As the condition progresses, it is not uncommon for people with moderate to advanced dementia to lose weight. It is often thought that weight loss is an inevitable part of the physical decline that accompanies advancing dementia. However, this is not the case probably until the end of life stage, which will be considered in Chapter 8. Weight loss usually results from a person simply not eating or drinking enough. This can sometimes be due to poor understanding of the person' needs and preferences for food and drink, and not ensuring they have an adequate intake. The consequences of low body weight can be serious because it increases the risk of a number of harmful conditions, including hypothermia, osteoporosis, fracture, depression, impaired immunity, delayed healing, pressure sores and micronutrient deficiencies. Alternatively, for some people, the problem may be overeating or inappropriate eating, such as eating too much of one type of food or trying to eat non-edible products due to poor recognition. As a person with moderate dementia often cannot meet their own nutritional needs, carers must take on that responsibility themselves.

What is an appropriate diet for an older person with moderate dementia? Overall, what is healthy for the rest of us is healthy for someone with dementia. However, it is generally better for older people to be slightly overweight than underweight, so if the person is experiencing weight loss a diet high in calories may be appropriate. Plenty of bread, cakes, potatoes, sugar, fats and chocolate may not be recommended for most of us but are just the ticket for an older person who is losing weight! Those caring for the person should consult their GP and advice from a dietician may be beneficial. As we suggested earlier, there is no reason why people with dementia should not enjoy alcoholic drinks in limited amounts, if that is what they have been used to. (We cannot recommend smoking but acknowledge that a person who has always smoked may experience enhanced well-being if allowed to continue to do so!)

DIFFICULTIES WITH EATING AND DRINKING

Moderate dementia may affect a person's ability to meet their nutritional needs in a number of ways, and those caring for the person should again use dementia empathy to appreciate why the person is having difficulties. Possible explanations for eating and drinking issues may include the following.

- Impaired recognition of food and drink: a person's memory and attention difficulties may lead them to simply not notice that food has been put in front of them, particularly if it has been placed beyond their immediate field of attention, or they may not recognise it as food. This might result from their being given something to eat that they are not used to, or that is not presented in a clear way.

- Loss of ability to express likes, dislikes and preferences: if a person is given a meal by someone who does not know them well, they may be given something they dislike but not be able to express their feelings clearly. It can also sometimes be the case that people with dementia sometimes come to dislike food that they previously enjoyed, perhaps due to their condition affecting their sense of taste.

- Impaired ability to concentrate on a meal: a person's memory and attention difficulties may make it hard for them to concentrate on a meal long enough to finish it. They may leave a meal half eaten and those caring for them will assume that they have had enough, but it could be that their attention has wandered. Sometimes a person who likes to walk about a lot may find it hard to sit still for long enough to eat a full meal.

- Impaired ability to use cutlery: impairment of executive function can affect a person's ability to use a knife and fork with proper skill, or to cut up food. Again this may result in their leaving food because they are unable to prepare it for eating.

- Impaired hand-mouth co-ordination: a person's ability to co-ordinate fine movements such as putting food into their mouth may also be impaired. They may drop food and not be able to retrieve it, or eat 'messily', becoming reluctant to finish their meal because of embarrassment.

HELPING A PERSON WITH MODERATE DEMENTIA MEET THEIR NUTRITIONAL NEEDS

As with other aspects of behaviour, understanding the reasons for that behaviour is the first step to finding creative solutions. In no particular order, we would offer the following suggestions for helping a person eat and drink properly.

- Know the person's accustomed eating habits: this is of course easier for those such as close family who know the person well. Despite the possibility of tastes changing, most people will enjoy best those foods that they have always preferred. Maintaining accustomed routines is also important, so that the person eats at times and in a place they are used to.

- Provide an environment conducive to eating and drinking: a distraction-free and relaxing environment will help the person concentrate on their meal and will reduce restlessness. Clear lighting and a minimum of extraneous noise are helpful. It may be better to leave the television off, if it appears that it is putting the person off; relaxing background music may be better.

- Promote attention to food: use the principles of dementia empathy to help the person recognise and attend to their meals. Food that is colourful and easily recognised is best. Ensure that they know that their meal is there by putting food and drink where they can see and recognise it, and orientating them to their meal verbally. Having a contrast between the plate and the table is helpful for visual-spatial difficulties – for example, having brightly coloured plates against a plain different coloured tablecloth, or having a visible rim round the edge of the plate. If the person appears to lose attention half way through their meal, it may be helpful to take it away for a little while, rearrange it on the plate so that it looks more presentable and then give it to the person again.

- Encourage and assist as necessary – but don't patronise: the person who has difficulties with using cutlery or with hand to mouth co-ordination may need some assistance with eating, but the principle should be to maintain their independence and dignity as much as possible. They should only be helped to eat if they really cannot manage themselves (see Chapter 7). Sometimes it will be appropriate to cut up their food so they can manage it better, or for them to use a spoon rather than a knife and fork. Alternatively, they may manage better with 'finger food' that they can pick up. As anyone who has organised a buffet party knows, there is a very wide range of tasty foods that can be served to be eaten without cutlery!

- Minimise constipation through high-fibre food, adequate hydration and promoting exercise: constipation is a frequent difficulty for people with dementia and it may make them reluctant to eat or restless through discomfort. Constipation can be minimised by including high-fibre foods, particularly vegetables and fruit, in a person's diet, by ensuring that they drink adequate fluids and by promoting exercise.

- Adopt a flexible approach if the person cannot concentrate on meals: sometimes it is better to make food available on a flexible basis if the person is too restless to concentrate on set mealtimes. Offer frequent snacks and drinks during the day that can be eaten easily if the person is walking about. Sometimes they will feel hungrier at night times, so making snacks available then may help settle a restless person.

- Monitor the person's weight: as stated earlier, weight loss can be serious so those caring for the person should keep their weight under review. Dementia does not in itself lead to weight loss, so if the person is losing weight it is for another reason. Often weight loss results from the eating problems discussed previously, but it is also possible that a person who walks about much of the time may lose weight because of the amount of exercise they are taking. In these cases, bulking up meals with extra carbohydrates may be appropriate. Weight loss may also reflect an underlying physical health problem that may require medical attention. Some people with moderate dementia may go through a phase of eating excessively and put on a great deal of weight, particularly if they are not active. This is a potential problem and those caring for the person should reduce portion sizes accordingly.

- Eating and drinking are activities! We should always remember that we eat and drink for enjoyment as much as (or more than) for nutritional reasons and we should help people with moderate dementia gain enjoyment from their meals. Make mealtimes pleasant occasions and opportunities for conversation and socialisation. A glass of wine or beer often adds a certain *je ne sais quoi* to a meal! And don't be afraid to eat out if that is something the person used to enjoy. Playing background music can also help add to the sense of enjoyment and relaxation.

- As dementia progresses to the advanced phase, other issues may occur such as swallowing difficulties and the person may become unable to feed themselves. We will address these issues in Chapter 7.

Meeting continence needs

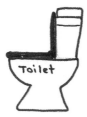

An inevitable consequence of eating and drinking is the need to go to the toilet and difficulties become more common as dementia progresses. Using the toilet is of course a taboo subject in most cultures, as well as often being a smelly and unpleasant one. People with dementia find difficulties with using the toilet as embarrassing and distressing as do family members and friends. Those with moderate dementia may have difficulties in meeting their needs to pass urine, or faeces, or both. Those caring for a person with moderate dementia will inevitably need to grasp the nettle of assisting the person with meeting their continence needs and how they do so will have a strong influence on the person's well-being and sense of dignity.

CAUSES OF DIFFICULTIES WITH USING THE TOILET

Broadly speaking, difficulties with using the toilet may result from three main causes:

- In the earlier phases of dementia, a person is aware of their need to go to the toilet and most of the time manages to meet their continence needs. However, growing memory, attention and executive function impairment may affect their ability to go to the toilet independently. A number of obstacles may present themselves in that a person may:

  ◆ not be able to express clearly that they need to go to the toilet, or to ask where the toilet is

  ◆ not be able to find their way to the toilet

- ◆ set off for the toilet but then forget where they were going

- ◆ leave it too late to get to the toilet

- ◆ may not be able to manage the toilet door

- ◆ find it difficult to adjust their clothing in time

- ◆ have difficulty actually using the toilet

- ◆ successfully use the toilet but then have difficulty in cleaning themselves and re-adjusting their clothing.

All these challenges may result in the person having an 'accident', with consequent embarrassment and possible bad feelings.

- A person's need to go to the toilet may be heightened by physical health issues. Urinary tract infections, stomach upsets, prostate problems in men and constipation can all lead to the person needing to go to the toilet more urgently than usual, leading to less time for the person to 'problem solve' using the toilet successfully.

- In the later phases of dementia, a person's awareness of their need to go to the toilet diminishes and eventually is lost. When this happens, the person becomes 'doubly incontinent'. We will consider this situation in Chapter 7.

'My wife started having problems with [faecal] continence; she seemed to be frightened of going to the toilet and was only going about once a fortnight. She had also started having problems finding the toilet. On one occasion she got into a terrible state and I eventually persuaded her and got her in the toilet and left her in there but when I went back the walls were covered, she was covered…it was awful.'

HELPING A PERSON WITH MODERATE DEMENTIA
MEET THEIR CONTINENCE NEEDS

This will challenge family members' and friends' qualities of tolerance and acceptance, but it is important that an open, accepting and non-blaming attitude is adopted if a person starts to have 'accidents'. Those caring for the person may need to take a proactive approach to helping them with using the toilet. Principles for assisting them to meet their needs will depend on their particular difficulties and may include the following.

- If the person has an accident, respond in an accepting and non-blaming way. Help them clean themselves and the mess up.

- Begin by trying to ascertain the actual difficulties that the person has. In the early and moderate phases of dementia, they may well be able to tell you what they feel the problem is. If not, observing them going to the toilet (embarrassing though that may be) may offer clues.

- If there is the possibility of a physical health cause (this may particularly be the case if the person suddenly starts having more accidents than usual), consult their GP.

- If the issue is that the person is inclined to forget about going to the toilet, it may be appropriate to tactfully remind them. Perhaps one could try saying something like, 'I'm dying for the loo, what about you?'

- Individual solutions are likely to be needed for the person's specific difficulties. If they can't find their way to the toilet, signs may help, or they may need to be shown the way. If they can't open the door, make sure it is left open. If managing clothing is the problem, then clothes that are easy to remove and put back on will help – the person can still wear things that are smart or stylish. Other issues may require imaginative approaches geared towards the individual's needs. In all cases an open, accepting but tactful and respectful manner on the part of family members and friends will help spare the person embarrassment and will maximise their ability to maintain independence in meeting their continence needs.

- In some cases, continence pads may be a practical solution to avoiding the embarrassment and inconvenience of accidents. Elasticated pull-up pads are available that may be helpful for people who are starting to lose control over their bladder or bowels. These look and feel like normal underpants, are easy to use and people with dementia usually tolerate them well. We will discuss the use of pads further in Chapter 7.

'My husband couldn't remember how to use the zip on his trousers so we chose tracksuit bottoms.'

Sleep disturbances

Disturbances in sleeping patterns are common among people with dementia and can become more of an issue in the moderate phase. This can be especially difficult for those living with the person who may also have their sleep disturbed. For people with dementia with Lewy bodies or Parkinson's disease, sleep disturbance can be particularly prevalent, but all types of dementia can affect sleeping.

CAUSES OF SLEEP DISTURBANCES

It is important to try and understand what may be causing the problem in order to decide which strategies might help. In the first instance, keeping a diary may be useful in establishing what the pattern is and what is happening to a person during the day. Factors that can contribute towards a disturbed sleep include:

- physical health problems such as urine infections or prostate problems, which may lead to an increased need to use the toilet

- pain or discomfort, including arthritis and leg cramps

- reduced need for sleep or sleeping too much during the day

- depression, which can cause early morning wakening

- environmental disturbances – for example, poor lighting, noise or inappropriate temperature

- nightmares

- restless leg syndrome or uncontrolled limb movements – these symptoms are commonly experienced by people with dementia with Lewy bodies or Parkinson's disease.

HELPING SOMEONE ACHIEVE A MORE SETTLED SLEEP PATTERN

While there may be no easy solution to sleep disturbances, it is essential that the possible causes are investigated so that those who are doing the caring can also get their much needed sleep. Going without sleep must be one of the most difficult things to cope with for all concerned and is likely to increase irritability for everyone. One of us is known for her love of sleep but also her short temper if she doesn't get enough of it! It is worth asking for a physical health check if there are any signs or symptoms of ill health that might be causing the sleep pattern of the person with dementia to be disturbed. Other suggestions derive from dementia empathy – like the rest of us, people with dementia need the right circumstances in order to get a good night's sleep.

- Try to establish a regular routine, if possible, that includes exercise in the morning, and avoid difficult tasks that may cause distress in the late afternoon or early evening.

- Ensure adequate light and activity during the day because this helps establish a good sleep pattern.

- Try to avoid long periods of sleep during the day.

- Avoid consumption of caffeine and alcohol in the evening.

- Consider whether medications are causing sleep problems – ACEI drugs can cause night-time stimulation and dream disturbance, so should not be taken in the evening.

- Check the temperature of the bedroom is comfortable: not too hot or too cold.

- Use low level or night lights to help the person find the bathroom and promote orientation.

- If the person is in an unfamiliar environment, try to put familiar things in sight such as photos or prized possessions.

- Play soft music as the person goes to sleep.

If the person continues to have disturbed sleep or refuses to go to bed at a reasonable time, then try to be flexible: let them sleep on the sofa or make sure the house is safe if they walk around in the night. It may be necessary for those who are caring to sleep in a separate bed or room, if possible, so that both people do not have a disturbed night.

Sleep disturbances may be a stage that the person with dementia goes through, which will subside and settle over time. As dementia progresses to the advanced phase, people tend to sleep more. If problems persist, then medical advice may be sought about night-time sedation, although this is generally not advised for people with dementia because of the risk of increased confusion. However, a short-term trial of sleeping tablets may help with re-establishing a routine, although this should be monitored carefully. Alternatively a trial of an anti-depressant may be offered, but again this should be monitored for any undesirable side effects such as sedation or dizziness.

SUNDOWNING

This is a term used to describe an increase in unsettled behaviour or restlessness that sometimes happens in the moderate stage of dementia, during late afternoon or early evening – in other words, when the sun is going down. While there is some debate about the exact nature of sundowning, it is thought to be caused by a disturbance in circadian rhythms due to changes in the brain and is often linked with sleep disturbance. This can be very distressing and especially as it occurs at a time when carers may want to 'wind down'. The principles used in helping people sleep better should be equally applied so that a person is encouraged to get plenty of light and activity earlier in the day; long periods of sleeping during the day are discouraged; and excessive noise and activity are reduced during late afternoon and early evening.

Professional support for people with moderate dementia, their families and friends

We discussed in Chapter 3 informal and professional support services for people with early dementia such as support groups, home care, day centres and respite care. Such services are likely to be of even greater value to those caring for people with moderate dementia – it is possible that families will not access help (or be regarded as needing help) until a person has reached this phase. A person with moderate dementia may need greater assistance with daily living than family members can readily provide, or they may have activity needs that can be met more effectively in day care settings. As the person's needs increase, different countries will have their own systems to determine what support can be offered and how this is paid for. An assessment of need will often take place to help work out what help the person with dementia requires. At this point it is essential that families are involved in the assessment so their views are included and they can help co-ordinate the care.

> 'All Grandma's appointments for services would be sent to her address, and she would open them and put them somewhere and we wouldn't know about them and I found it so frustrating, it seemed obvious to me, why would you send appointments to a person who has dementia when they're not necessarily going to remember to pass them on?'

Specialist services for people with dementia may be available such as community nurses or specially trained staff who can provide direct care or respite at home. Although specialist services are increasing in some areas, they are still not widely available in most countries. On the whole, care will often be provided by untrained staff who may or may not understand about dementia and, while there are also many skilful and empathic carers, it can sometimes be a challenge ensuring the person has the right support.

> 'Introducing the carer was very difficult as my wife didn't want any help; the first person didn't work as my wife didn't like her. However when Mary started it worked well from the beginning. My wife didn't like to upset people but Mary was very skilled and did things like going shopping with my wife; made her feel included. This was such a relief. It took a few weeks before they settled in but eventually my wife thought she was lovely.'

It is the expertise and knowledge of family and friends that is vital in ensuring that care is provided that meets the individual needs of the person. Information such as that collected in life stories should be shared with professionals, and family or friends should not be shy to point out tactfully if they see care is not being provided in an inappropriate way. At the same time, for family members or friends who may be responsible for a lot of hands-on care at this stage, getting support from professionals is essential both in terms of advice and emotional support and also in order to have a break from caring.

The other main professional service for people with moderate dementia is residential care. Many families sooner or later take the considerable step of seeking a care home place for the person they have been looking after. We will consider the issues around residential care in the next chapter.

When people with dementia are admitted to hospital

As the majority of people with dementia are older people and therefore more prone to physical illness, it follows that a person with dementia may at some time be admitted to a general hospital. As dementia itself may make the person more vulnerable to physical conditions, the numbers are high: in the UK, for example, approximately 25 per cent of all general hospital beds at any time are occupied by people with dementia and probably more if dementia were properly recognised and diagnosed (Alzheimer's Society 2009). In this section we will consider the issues facing people with dementia, their families and friends, if a person is admitted to a general hospital (we won't in this section discuss care of people with dementia who are reaching the end of life – this will be addressed in Chapter 8).

WHAT LEADS TO PEOPLE WITH DEMENTIA BEING ADMITTED TO HOSPITAL?

The most common reasons for admission to general hospital are:

- a fractured hip following a fall

- a urinary tract infection (UTI)

- a chest infection (including pneumonia)

- a stroke

- a general failure to thrive, including loss of weight or self-neglect.

These conditions are common in older people but people with dementia may be particularly likely to experience them. Infections and other conditions may lead to a person experiencing delirium (see Chapter 2), which may lead to a temporary rise in 'confusion', disorientation and memory difficulties – people with dementia are particularly prone to episodes of delirium when physically unwell.

The risk of a person developing these conditions may be reduced if they are well looked after, well nourished and exercise regularly (but safely, to avoid falls). If they do experience infections such as UTIs or pneumonia, these may be treatable in their home or care home setting and there is evidence that GPs refer people with dementia to hospital too readily, without properly considering community-based treatment and care.

ISSUES FOR PEOPLE WITH DEMENTIA
IN GENERAL HOSPITALS

Avoiding unnecessary hospital admission is important because there is strong evidence that people with dementia do not fare well in general hospitals. People with dementia spend longer in hospital, recover less quickly and effectively and have higher mortality rates than people of similar ages and conditions who do not have dementia. A period in hospital may lead to a person entering residential care prematurely as a result of poor recovery. The person may lack awareness of the fact that they are ill and may well not co-operate with treatment. Furthermore, general hospitals are not good environments for people with dementia. Hospital wards are noisy, unfamiliar and confusing places that are rarely conducive to their needs. It can also be difficult for people with dementia to walk about safely in a hospital ward or to find their way around. People with dementia may be unable to find their way to the toilet on a hospital ward or to ask staff for help, leading to an increased frequency of accidents. Small wonder that many people with dementia experience increased distress and anxiety, further compromising their recovery.

Another factor that can affect recovery in general hospitals is that staff can be unprepared for caring for people with dementia. Our own research has shown that many general nurses receive little or no training about caring for people with dementia. A particular issue is eating and drinking. General hospital staff can sometimes be unaware that a person's cognitive difficulties can compromise their ability to give themselves adequate nourishment, and therefore don't offer appropriate assistance. Lack of understanding among staff of appropriate ways of interacting with people with dementia or responding to behaviour that they find difficult can lead to excessive use of sedative medication – further compromising the person's physical health. Difficulties faced by staff in general hospitals include inadequate staffing levels and the fact that the focus of care is often 'fast paced' and geared towards acute illness rather than long-term conditions such as dementia.

Surveys of family carers and people with dementia in the UK reveal the following concerns about care and treatment in general hospitals (Thompson and Heath 2011) and similar issues have been raised in other countries:

- Nurses not recognising or understanding dementia.

- Staff not having enough time to provide good care.

- Lack of person-centred care and individualised care plans.

- A person not being helped to eat or drink.

- Lack of opportunity for social interaction.

- Not as much opportunity for involvement in decision making as wished for (for patient as well as family).

- Poor communication with families.

- A person being moved too frequently between different wards.

- Unsuitable environments.

It is recognised that improving general hospital care and working to avoid admissions that are not necessary are important ways to improve the experience for people with dementia and their families. One of us carried out investigations into hospital care that highlighted that attention to improving the understanding of staff, enhancing assessment and recognition of dementia, involving families in care, changing the environment and making care individualised are all important ways in which care can be improved.

HOW CAN FAMILY MEMBERS AND FRIENDS HELP?

The ways that family members and friends can help improve the experience of people with dementia in general hospitals are similar to their contribution if a person receives residential care, and we will discuss these principles in Chapter 6. Essentially, families and friends can assist by telling hospital staff about the person, their past life (so that staff have a better appreciation of them as individuals), their likes and dislikes and any tips or strategies for assisting with aspects of care. It may in some cases be appropriate to give actual assistance with things such as eating and drinking or helping the person use the toilet. Spending time with the person and doing activities will help relieve boredom and distress. Above all, there is no intrinsic reason why people with dementia should not recover from physical illness as well as other people of the same age and circumstances, and family members and friends may sometimes need to be assertive with hospital staff to ensure that appropriate care standards are maintained.

Vulnerability and abuse

It will be clear that because of their lack of mental capacity people with moderate dementia are particularly vulnerable to the risk of coming to harm in that their ability to understand their situation, make rational decisions and look after themselves will all be significantly impaired. We have discussed situations where the person may come to harm as a result of their own actions, but we must also be aware that people with dementia may be at risk of harm from others – including those who are in a caring relationship with the person, such as family members, friends and professional carers. A number of types of abuse may be identified:

- Physical abuse: we will all surely agree that, if one hits, kicks or slaps a person with dementia, then one has abused that person. Furthermore, if one acted in this way towards an older person, the harm caused could be disproportionately greater if the person were physically frail.

- Psychological abuse: within this category are included threats of harm or abandonment, deprivation of contact, humiliation, blaming, controlling, intimidation, coercion, harassment and verbal abuse. Some of these have echoes of Tom Kitwood's categories of malignant social psychology, discussed in Chapter 4 (Kitwood 1997). Cynics might say that they are also part and parcel of many interpersonal encounters and even many relationships. But as we discussed earlier, people with dementia may be particularly affected by such things, because they are likely to lack the wherewithal to defend themselves or answer back.

- Sexual abuse: this includes rape and sexual assault, or sexual acts to which the vulnerable adult has not consented, or could not consent, or was pressured into consenting. We may feel that sexual abuse of older people in general and people with dementia in particular is very unlikely to happen – but not many years ago it was widely believed that sexual abuse of children rarely happened as well. Nowadays we recognise how relatively common child sexual abuse is and it could be that in years to come we will discover that sexual abuse of older people is also widespread. It certainly does happen, as occasional reports of court cases prove.

- Financial or material abuse: this includes theft, fraud, exploitation, pressure in connection with wills, property or inheritance, or financial transactions, or the misuse or misappropriation of property, possessions or benefits. People with dementia are especially vulnerable to financial abuse, particularly if they have built up savings. Research suggests that financial exploitation of older people by their own families is depressingly common. Anyone who has attempted to acquire power of attorney for a person with dementia will know how complex the application process is, largely to try to safeguard the person against exploitation. Others may of course exploit people with dementia financially because a person's reduced capacity for decision making may cause them to make unwise financial arrangements. Unscrupulous individuals may 'befriend' a person with the intention of getting money from them and we are also familiar with news reports of tradesmen or doorstep salespersons who charge extortionate fees for services that a person does not need.

- Neglect and acts of omission: this includes ignoring medical or physical care needs, failure to provide access to appropriate health or social care services and the withholding of the necessities of life, such as medication, adequate nutrition or heating. We have discussed earlier how people with moderate dementia rely on others to meet their daily living needs, and the complexities that may arise in helping people with dementia meet those needs. Again, failure by those caring for a person with dementia to fulfil their caring responsibilities is sadly not uncommon.

- Discriminatory abuse: this is perhaps an unexpected category but it is nevertheless an important one when considering people with dementia. It embraces comments or actions that are racist, sexist or based on a person's disability, and other forms of harassment, slurs or similar treatment. People with dementia may be on the receiving end of racial or sexual slurs, as may the rest of us and, as stated earlier, may lack the ability to make an appropriate response. In addition, they may also experience discrimination as a result of having dementia. We have observed that the public's view of dementia, reflected in the media, is a negative one and people with dementia are often described in pejorative terms – 'gaga', 'gone back to childhood', etc. We have also heard of people with dementia who have been refused access to pubs and restaurants on account of their condition.

WHAT CAN FAMILY MEMBERS AND FRIENDS DO IF THEY SUSPECT THAT A PERSON WITH DEMENTIA IS BEING ABUSED?

This is a difficult question to answer. The nature of dementia of course means that the person is unlikely to be able to complain that they are being abused, or if they do so they may not be believed. It is also possible that they may not be aware that abuse is taking place. Also, families are complicated entities and interfering with longstanding relationships, even if those relationships appear to be dysfunctional, may not necessarily be in the person's best interests. At the same time, one should not stand back and let a person with dementia suffer abuse or neglect – it is not unknown for older people to die as a result. Discussions within the family may help, or concerned individuals could contact their local authority. Charities exist to offer confidential advice (for example, Action on Elder Abuse in the UK) and if it is felt that the situation is serious then the police should be contacted – abusing or neglecting a vulnerable adult is potentially a criminal offence.

CHAPTER 6

The Decision

Considering Residential Care for People with Dementia

Perceptions of residential care

Some of us who were brought up with British television will remember a classic sketch by the great comedians Morecambe and Wise. Eric Morecambe says something silly and the stern 'straight man' Ernie Wise puts him right with a long lecture about Eric's inadequacies and how he, Ernie, has had enough of looking after him. In response, Morecambe puts on a mock-pathetic face and in a small voice says, 'Are you going to put me in a home?'

The line raises a laugh because of the absurdity of the idea and Eric Morecambe's comic genius. At the same time, it hits a nerve in that it taps into our beliefs and stereotypes about residential care. Such care often receives negative press coverage and we may hold significant concerns about whether it is right for our loved ones. Sometimes our concerns about residential care are well founded. Sadly, stories of drab, unstimulating, neglectful and sometimes downright abusive care homes crop up from time to time. However, there is nothing inevitable about the notion that residential care equals bad care. Many care homes today are bright, welcoming, well-run establishments, with staff who are skilled in dementia care and have residents' best interests at heart. For some people with moderate dementia, going to live in a care home can be a positive experience that enhances their well-being and quality of life.

This is not to say that all people who reach a certain point in the journey through dementia should as a matter of course go to live in a care home. The decision to seek residential care for a person with dementia is a complex and often difficult one, and every family will need to make that decision through a close consideration of individual circumstances. It is also the case that not all care homes are alike. The decision of where a person should live can be as hard as the decision to seek residential care in the first place. In this section we will consider some of the many factors that families must take into account in making these decisions. We will also consider how families and friends can maintain relationships with the person once they are living in residential care.

What is residential care?

Residential care facilities are places where some people with dementia live. Different countries use different terms and residential care is organised in different ways but the basic principle is the same. In the UK the term 'care home' is now used to cover any formal setting where people live and are looked after by paid staff, but you may still hear the terms 'nursing home' and 'residential home'. In the USA a number of terms are used, including 'nursing home' and 'dementia care units' and in Canada they also talk about 'nursing homes' or 'homes for the aged'. Finally, in Australia the term currently in use is 'aged care home (high or low level)'. Given the complexity and variation of terminology, for convenience we will use the UK term 'care home' in this section and the rest of the book.

Care homes are in essence hotels that in addition to a bedroom, meals and leisure facilities provide a measure of personal or nursing care for residents. Some care homes are specifically approved for people with dementia, but people with dementia can be found elsewhere within residential care settings. In the UK, as in many English-speaking and European countries, care homes are largely owned and managed by private companies rather than by the government. Companies vary greatly in size, from large national concerns that own hundreds of homes to independent providers that may own just one or two. Payment arrangements for people living in care homes can be complex but often the person themselves (or their family on their behalf) must pay some or all of the costs, depending on their savings and assets.

Research shows that the majority of older people want to live in their own homes, or with their families, rather than in care homes, and surveys of family carers indicate that this is what they would prefer as well. It is understandable that people would want if possible to live in surroundings that are private and familiar and with their families rather than with strangers. The negative image of care homes that we discussed earlier also undoubtedly contributes to the preference for staying at home. In addition, residential care is expensive, both for individuals and for governments that must fund those who cannot pay for themselves. According to Alzheimer's Disease International, in most high income countries it is estimated that only one-third of people with dementia live in care homes, despite sometimes having extensive care needs and in middle or low income countries only 5 per cent will be afforded this kind of support. As a commentator succinctly if rather cynically put it, 'Most people with dementia live at home, this is where they want to live, this is where their families want them to live, and this is where the government wants them to live' (Graham 2003).

The decision

There are many families and friends who continue to care for people with dementia throughout the progression of the person's condition, and we will discuss some of the principles of caring for people with advanced dementia in the next chapter. At the same time, we believe that in some situations a care home may be the best place for the person to live and families and friends should not feel guilty about taking that step. Furthermore, we believe that living in a care home will not necessarily lead to the person experiencing a poorer quality of life and sense of well-being, and good care homes (like good hotels) can be pleasant, stimulating and enjoyable places. In short, a move to a care home may indeed be the best thing for the person and their families and friends.

> 'I was encouraged by the social worker to start having a look at nursing homes just to see what was out there; this was very traumatic but I went to have a look at a few places; on reflection it helped prepare me.'

In order for this outcome to be achieved, however, families and friends must think through the issues and plan for the move carefully. Sometimes this is not possible, if the move comes about as a result of a crisis situation, such as a sudden deterioration in the person's health, or the health of their main carer. In most cases, though, a move to a care home will have been considered more or less openly for some time. This leads to a rather important question.

SHOULD THE PERSON WITH DEMENTIA BE INVOLVED IN THE DECISION?

Part of our own fear of residential care may be that we will be 'put away' without being able to do anything about it. But is it possible to meaningfully consult a person with dementia about moving to a care home if they are in a moderate or advanced stage of dementia? The concern may be that the person will either not understand what is being suggested to them or will immediately say 'no', either because they do not want to leave their home or because they believe that their ability to live at home is greater than their family's estimation. Many family members and friends will understandably avoid including the person in the decision for these reasons.

In some cases, however, it may be possible that the person can have some say. As we discussed in Chapter 3, a person may make an advanced decision about aspects of their future care and that decision may include a statement about what the person would want to happen if living at home became difficult. It is not uncommon for people to say they would not want to become a 'burden' to their families. The person might in effect give permission for family and friends to seek residential care for them in certain circumstances and may express preferences about where they would like to live. Even if the person has reached the phase of moderate dementia, we should not assume that the question cannot be discussed with them. They may retain enough awareness to understand the implications of what is being proposed and may not necessarily disagree with the proposal, recognising at some level that such a move may be for the best. As we will see later, the transition to residential care may be easier if the person has been prepared as far as possible for the move. However, sometimes the decision has to be taken by families and friends in the person's best interests and without their consent, or even their awareness, and families should not feel guilty about taking this step.

> 'We're past the point where Grandma can participate in any decisions. I know she wants to stay at home but…'

MAKING THE DECISION

The decision-making process will be different for each family and will be easier for some than for others. As suggested earlier, sometimes the decision will in effect be taken out of their hands, if the person's main carer (who may well be an elderly spouse or partner) becomes ill or even dies and no one else is able to take on the caring role. In such cases an emergency admission to hospital is often the first step to the person's inevitable move to a care home, although this is not desirable. The decision may be more or less straightforward if the person has previously indicated their willingness to live in a care home.

For others, the decision is far from easy and again the nature of the relationship is likely to be a predominant factor. A husband or wife may not want to be parted from their life partner or an adult child may feel massive guilt about giving up caring for their parent. Other family members may exert subtle pressure on the main carer's sense of duty and cultural factors may come into play as well. The person themselves may give out the message that they want to stay at home, sometimes by acting in a dependent way towards their main carer or expressing themselves in an agitated fashion when not at home, thereby adding to the carer's sense of responsibility. Family members, rightly or wrongly, may feel that they are condemning the person to a life of unhappiness or worse if they enter a care home. They may feel that nurses and paid carers cannot possibly know the person as well as their family does and will not be able to care as effectively and sensitively.

> 'Dementia, by its nature, presents a series of losses over time. The biggest loss was actually when my husband went in the care home. For the first time we were living apart, it felt like a death, but a line hadn't been drawn under it and you feel very bereaved.'

On the other hand, there is the fact that caring for a person with moderate dementia can be difficult and sometimes stressful and exhausting. Researchers talk about the burden of caring that family members and friends must sometimes bear. As we saw in Chapter 5, the person's manner and actions may cause difficulties for their carers. Helping the person with activities of daily living such as dressing, nutrition and keeping clean can be tiring. Sometimes the person's actions may put themselves or others at risk of harm and maintaining vigilance can be exhausting for carers. It may be particularly difficult and distressing for families and friends if the person is finding it hard to meet their toilet needs and this can be the 'straw that breaks the camel's back'.

Carers must also cope with the emotional aspects of caring – seeing a person they have known and loved for years changing in front of them and sometimes not appreciating what is being done for them. They may well also have to manage changes in other relationships. As we have discussed previously, family tensions can be exacerbated by caring and friendships can sometimes be broken when friends stop visiting. Adult children may have given up work in order to care, or will have no time for hobbies or interests. It is unsurprising that research has shown that carers of people with dementia report more burden (physical, emotional and financial) than those in other caring roles and have greater rates of common physical and mental health problems than those of similar ages and backgrounds who do not have a caring role.

For some the benefits of maintaining the caring role outweigh the drawbacks. Their emotional ties to the person with dementia may be strong enough for them to cope with the burden, or their support network may sustain them. Some people do not regard the caring role as especially burdensome at all – they get a sense of satisfaction and purpose from caring and continue to look after the person at home long after they would qualify for residential care. For many others, however, the point is reached when the sense of burden becomes too great, or the sheer practicalities of caring become too difficult, even with professional help. Then the decision is made, ideally with the contribution and support of other family members and friends and in conjunction with advice from professionals such as social workers or the person's GP, but sometimes alone.

'I'd like my husband to stay at home for as long as possible but I'm not going to be a martyr about it, if it came to the point that he needed more care than I can give him.'

'My sisters and I could see that Dad was getting tired but he would never say it was getting too much. We could see he was struggling so we got the social worker to come to the house for a meeting with us and she put it to Dad about Mum going into permanent residential care. He got upset and started to cry and said he didn't want to feel he'd given up on her.'

'It is a really hard thing to take in, just the thought of consigning my wife to the care of an institution. That's not what you commit to or get married for… You never expect to do this.'

'Although I got a lot of support from others I felt guilty – I felt like a "rotter". It helped that others were supportive of the decision to consider a care home and kept stressing that it was a personal decision; that there was no wrong and no right.'

Choosing a care home

In the large majority of cases family members and friends have a measure of choice regarding where the person with dementia goes to live. The responsibility of making this choice is considerable and can add to the stress of families already feeling guilty about making the move. The factors involved in making the choice will differ, with some families placing greater weight on particular aspects than others. In this section we will attempt to guide families and friends through the issues of selecting a care home on behalf of a person with dementia.

HOW TO FIND OUT ABOUT CARE HOMES

There are a huge number of care homes in countries such as the UK. Local authorities will keep lists or the information may be found in the local library or on the internet. Basic information that families and friends need includes the following.

- The owning company – is it a large or small concern?
- Will the home meet the person's needs? What level of nursing care does it provide, and does it have a specialised dementia care facility?
- What are the fees? Is the home affordable?
- Is it a large home divided into several units or a small single-unit facility?
- How many beds does the home have?

- Where is the home situated? Is it easy for families and friends to visit?

- Will the person have their own room?

- Does the home have grounds and gardens?

- Does written material about the home state that activities are provided?

This kind of basic information will be available from a home's website or brochure but of course says nothing about the quality of the home and the care it offers. Families and friends must use other sources of information regarding these aspects. Social workers or other professionals may be unable to offer their own opinions, so families and friends must find out in other ways.

- Personal recommendation: in many aspects of life, recommendations from trusted people are often the best way of ascertaining the quality of services, and care homes are no different. It will be the case, however, that only a minority of families will know someone who is already living in a home so other sources of information will be required. Internet sites are starting to be developed in which individuals post online their opinions of care homes, and such sites may become important sources of personal recommendations in the future.

- Official reports: in the UK the Care Quality Commission (CQC) inspects and approves care homes and their reports are available on the internet. Other countries will have similar systems. However, these reports only offer impressions based on sometimes brief inspection visits and they sometimes don't discuss a home in any detail.

- Visiting the home and talking to staff: just as we would not buy a house without viewing it, we should not decide upon a place for a person with dementia to live without visiting it and looking around. We would recommend that several homes are visited to build up a broad impression of what is available locally and to make comparisons. No care home is perfect and there may still be difficulties lurking under the surface, but much can be ascertained from a carefully planned and conducted visit.

What should be expected of a care home?

Family members and friends will get the best out of a visit to a care home by both talking to staff and looking around to observe the environment and the people – staff and residents – within it. The fundamental questions that one is attempting to answer are straightforward:

- Will the person be known, understood and treated as an individual? Will the staff have an attitude of respect and of wanting the best for their residents? Will they know their residents, not just as they are in the present but in the context of their past lives? Will the care they give be fitted to the needs of each individual? What is being looked for is evidence of what the psychologist Tom Kitwood (1997) and others have termed 'person-centred care'.

- Will the person with dementia be looked after well? A baseline standard is that residents should be clean, well dressed and properly nourished with food and fluids. However this must go hand-in-hand with other aspects of care: psychological, social and spiritual, and there must be evidence that the home's staff are proactive in promoting these aspects as well as providing a good standard of physical care.

- Will the person have a good quality of life? As we have been maintaining throughout this book, a good quality of life for people with dementia should embrace opportunities for interaction with others and meaningful activity. We may also add the opportunity to experience different environments, including access to the open air.

- Will the person experience a reasonable measure of well-being? While well-being cannot be guaranteed for any of us all the time, the sense of well-being of a person with dementia will be enhanced and maintained if the factors set out here are in place and if the care home staff take proper steps to assist the person if they are in some way distressed.

- Will families and friends be similarly respected? Family members and friends will have their own needs for information and support once a person goes to live in a care home and may also have a lot to offer the home's staff in terms of understanding the person and advice regarding aspects of care. Many will still want to be involved in the care of the person and a good care home will embrace the principles of 'relationship-based care' – regarding family members and friends as partners in caring for residents.

In seeking to achieve these aims, care home staff must show that they do *not* display what Tom Kitwood (1997) termed a 'standard paradigm' approach to people with dementia. Evidence of this includes the following.

- Staff displaying negative attitudes towards residents or a lack of sensitivity towards their needs. Sometimes this includes staff cutting corners or organising their working day to suit themselves rather than residents.

- Staff who concern themselves with physical or daily living care only, ignoring the social, psychological or spiritual sides of care. Along with this goes a lack of knowledge of residents as individuals.

- Care regimes that are 'one size fits all' rather than being individualised, with an over-reliance on routines and a lack of flexibility.

- An over-reliance on sedating medication (or even physical restraint) as a response to behaviour that staff find difficult, rather than staff trying to understand that behaviour and find creative ways of meeting the person's underlying needs.

- Family members and friends being ignored, patronised or excluded, and questions or complaints not taken seriously.

When visiting a home, families and friends should be trying to gauge to what extent care in the home reflects an underlying philosophy of person-centred rather than standard paradigm care. As stated earlier, no care home is perfect and the challenges that people with moderate or advanced dementia present will inevitably make it hard to support well-being at times. Also, resources will be limited in all but the most expensive care homes, leading to further compromises in the delivery of care. However, the ideals of person-centred care are no more than any of us would want or expect and so evidence should be present that the balance of care in a home is skewed much more towards the 'person-centred' end of the continuum and away from the 'standard paradigm' end.

Visiting a care home

When visiting a care home one is trying to make a judgement about where on our continuum the home lies. While it is very difficult to do this precisely, by taking note of some important aspects families and friends can gain as clear an idea as possible regarding the home and the likely quality of care it offers to residents.

TALK TO THE MANAGER

Much research has shown that the manager of any kind of care facility, whether it is a hospital ward or a care home, is crucial for setting the tone of that facility and marking out the quality standards expected of staff. Make sure you talk to the home manager and, if the home has a number of separate units, the manager of the unit where the person would live. Ask them about their philosophy of care and what they want for their residents.

Look for key words in their answer such as person-centred care, quality of life and well-being. Ask them also how they ensure that their staff fulfil that philosophy – a good manager will spend time on the 'shop floor' working directly with staff and residents. If the manager shows you around, look for how they talk to staff and residents while they do so: can you see evidence of mutual respect? Find out their views on the use of medication when residents act in ways that others find difficult. And if the manager is 'too busy' to see you, don't bother visiting.

FIND OUT ABOUT THE STAFF

Ask about the staff – numbers, qualifications, experience and specific training in dementia care. Ask to be introduced to some staff members. As you go around, look at what the staff are doing. Are they interacting with the residents or are they huddled together in the staff office? What is the quality of the interaction – is it respectful and person-centred?

TRY TO JUDGE RESIDENTS' WELL-BEING

Again as you go around, take note of what residents are doing and how contented they seem to be. Are they clean and presentable and do they appear to be well nourished? Do they seem to be distressed? Are they alert and active? If a high proportion of residents are asleep during the day, this may suggest an unstimulating environment or over-use of sedative medication. If residents have advanced dementia and physical frailty (see Chapter 7), are they comfortable? Is it apparent that staff have taken steps to get to know residents as people and to maintain their sense of individuality? Ask how staff find out about residents' previous lives and see if residents have personal belongings and things important to their identity such as family photographs and life story profiles.

LOOK FOR EVIDENCE OF ACTIVITIES

Ask about the provision of social and recreational activities and look for evidence that they are actually taking place. Most good homes will employ an activity co-ordinator, but ideally all staff should be involved in activities. Are residents taking part in activities during your visit or is it apparent that activities actually take place? Is it evident that residents have the opportunity to exercise out of doors?

WHAT IS THE PHYSICAL ENVIRONMENT LIKE?

Is the home's design and environment likely to promote well-being in people with dementia? Look for evidence that principles of dementia empathy have guided the development of the physical environment. Are the lights bright but not glaring? Have attempts been made to help residents maintain orientation, such as clear signs to toilets and bedrooms? Is extraneous noise minimised? Is there space where residents can walk about safely? Are there communual areas but also enough space so that residents don't feel crowded out by each other? Is the decor and furniture homely and in good condition? Are residents' rooms comfortable and personalised? Are there pictures on the walls and are they likely to be of interest to residents? Can you see evidence of objects that support activity such as games, books, music or occupational tools?

WHAT IS THE HOME'S ATTITUDE TOWARDS FAMILIES AND FRIENDS?

Put this question to the manager. A good home will welcome families and friends and will not restrict their visiting. Furthermore, a good home will encourage them to participate in care giving and will show concern for their needs (see later). Ask the manager if this is the case. If possible, ask to speak to relatives of residents, if any happen to be visiting.

JUDGE THE HOME'S 'FEEL'

We have visited many care homes over the years and sometimes it is possible to pick up the ambience of a home as soon as one walks through the front door. Some 'feel' good and others don't. Little things may come together to create a positive or negative 'feel'. Smell is an obvious indicator. With doubly incontinent residents some smell of urine or faeces may be inevitable, but if that smell hits strongly as soon as you walk in, that may be a sign that staff have been leaving residents in a soiled state for too long. Noise is another sign – is there a lot of shouting out by residents (or even by staff)? A subtle trick is to listen to what station the radio is tuned to – if it is blaring out pop music, it is likely that young care staff have tuned it to a channel that they want to listen to, rather than one that is appropriate for residents. Does the home appear to be a lively place – are there plants and pets and even dolls and toys? How welcoming or otherwise are staff when they see you – do they have good 'front of house' skills? At the end of the day, a good care home will be like a good hotel – welcoming, relaxing, quiet and efficient, with evidence that the staff value their residents and want the best for them.

Making the transition

The transition from living at home to living in a care home may well not be easy for either the person with dementia or their family. Proper preparation will help to make the transition as smooth as possible.

INVOLVING THE PERSON IN THE MOVE

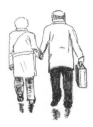

We pointed out earlier that some families do not ask or tell the person with dementia of their intention to seek a residential care place, thinking that the person will either not understand or will resist the idea. While this approach may be understandable, it can make the transition more difficult. Broaching the subject may, however, be problematic if the person's cognitive difficulties are such that they cannot understand the concept of a care home. It is a good idea for the person themselves to visit the homes on the family's shortlist along with the family carer (this should be after the family has made a first exploratory visit), to see if they appear to like and feel settled in each home. How this is introduced to the person will depend on circumstances; some will go along with the family willingly while others may be suspicious of where they are going. Families have been known to resort to telling the person things like, 'We're going out for a drive and we'll call in somewhere for tea.'

> 'I spoke to my wife about it and I told her that I had spoken to the doctor and that she needed to go into a clinic; she was happy with this.'

MAKING THE MOVE

Sooner or later the choice of home will be made and arrangements for the move put into place. Sometimes the person will go for a trial period, to see if they settle in the home and it meets their needs; in other cases, a clean transition is made. Families and friends can ease the transition by keeping the person as aware of events as possible, by trying not to appear distressed themselves and by working with the home's staff to help the person settle in. Co-ordinating the move with staff is important. The person should be expected and welcomed by the home's staff, shown around and helped with their belongings. Familiar clothes and objects will help relieve their anxieties and suspicions and family members can help them unpack and put things away in their room (again, some people with dementia may believe they are staying at a hotel and it may be helpful for them to do so). When saying goodbye, again maintain a calm and reassuring manner and tell the person you will be back to see them soon.

> 'I took my wife into her room; the carers came in and they were lovely and they said to me that the best thing was that I should go. She looked a little bit concerned but was OK.'

> 'There was a lot of wrench; you still care about the person but you are not in control.'

Staying involved

When a person with dementia goes to live in a care home, it does not mean that family members and friends have no further role to play, though sadly a minority will either visit infrequently or stop having any contact with the person at all. For the majority, however, moving to a care home simply begins a new phase in the caring journey. Family carers will have mixed feelings. On the one hand, they will feel a measure of relief that some of their sense of burden has been lifted and they have more freedom for other aspects of their lives. Indeed, as one carer said: 'When my mum went into a home it allowed me to be a daughter again and it improved our relationship.' On the other hand, many will feel a sense of loss, especially if the person with dementia is their spouse or partner, and they may well also experience ongoing feelings of guilt at instigating the move, particularly if the person does not appear to be settled in their new home. The majority of family members and friends want to stay involved in the person's care and a good care home will assist them to do so.

'I say to people that I am still a carer, just because I am not providing for my wife 24 hours a day doesn't mean that I don't care. I still make key decisions.'

HELPING THE TRANSITION

As suggested earlier, one way that families and friends can contribute to a person's care is by giving the care home staff information and advice about the person in order to help them get to know them better and care for them more effectively. It is important that a person with dementia is understood in the context of the whole of their life, so that staff can appreciate and respect the person as an individual and understand aspects of their actions and manner in terms of their biography. Many care homes compile more or less comprehensive life histories of new residents (see Chapter 3) and family members and friends are clearly the main sources of information for these exercises. Good care home staff are also open to ideas from families and friends regarding aspects of caring for the person and will welcome hints and strategies that family members can pass on based on their own experience of caring for the person. As we have also suggested, bringing in personal belongings, mementoes and photographs (and also perhaps recordings of favourite music that staff can play to the person) will help the person settle and maintain their sense of identity.

VISITING

Clearly the main way that family members and friends can stay involved is by visiting the person. Many people with moderate dementia will continue to recognise their loved ones even if they have little awareness of other aspects of their surroundings, and they will 'light up' when familiar people arrive. Even if the person's condition has progressed so much that they no longer appear to know even those closest to them, visits will enhance the person's well-being (see Chapter 7). There are no hard and fast rules about how frequent visits should be; a few family members may visit every day but all visits are valuable.

> 'The staff made a fuss of my dad as he visited Mum every day; they'd make him his lunch and they were always very welcoming to him.'

> 'My wife seemed to accept where she was and we visited every day; she has never asked how long she would be in for or ever asked to come home.'

Visits can provide extra opportunities for activity as well as conversation and, if the person's language ability is impaired, then spending the time carrying out an activity may be more fruitful (see Chapter 4 for ideas). Good care homes will encourage families and friends to take residents out and will enable them to get involved in activities within the home.

Family members and friends can also assist with daily living activities. Good homes allow visitors to stay during mealtimes and some family members enjoy helping the person eat their meals. Many people with dementia like to dress up and look their best and again visitors can sometimes assist in this area.

> 'If when I visit, my wife's not good I go away feeling terrible but when she's happy I feel OK. I have spoken to other carers who say they feel the same.'

Issues with residential care

We hope we have painted a positive picture of residential care in this chapter. There are many care homes with skilled, committed and empathic staff, and many people with dementia live lives in homes that are of good quality and promote well-being. It is, however, the case that issues can arise with residential care and we will outline some of the more common ones here.

WHEN THE PERSON DOES NOT SETTLE

As discussed earlier, good practice by care home staff in co-operation with families and friends will maximise the chances of the person with dementia settling into their new home. Sometimes, however, this does not appear to happen. The person may appear to be distressed and agitated and may make frequent attempts to leave the home. Some may react aggressively to staff, particularly if they do not approach the person in a sensitive way. In extreme circumstances, the care home manager will decide that the person cannot stay at the home and in most cases this is their prerogative.

This situation should be avoided by careful selection of a home, including family members being honest with the home staff about the person's manner and actions and a well-managed transition period. Clearly a move to another home (sometimes preceded by an emergency hospital admission) is highly disruptive for the person, who may become even more unsettled following subsequent moves, but it should be acknowledged that occasionally this will occur.

In most cases the person will eventually settle and families and friends can aid this process by working with the staff to come up with an individualised care plan for them. Sometimes this may involve families and friends visiting more frequently, or it may involve less frequent visits if all agree that this will be in the person's best interests. Legal procedures may need to be gone through to ensure the person's safety by giving staff the legal right to prevent them from leaving the home.

YOUNGER PEOPLE WITH DEMENTIA IN RESIDENTIAL CARE

We discussed the specific issues related to younger people with dementia in Chapter 1. A proportion of those under the age of 60 who have dementia will require residential care. This can create issues because the numbers of such people in a given geographical area are likely to be very small and specialist residential care facilities are unlikely to be available. This means that younger people must often go to live in care homes that normally cater for much older residents. This can be awkward for the person, who must live with people considerably older than themselves. It can also create challenges for staff because the person may be physically fitter and more active than other residents, may not appreciate the same activities as older residents and may have particular care needs if they have an uncommon form of dementia. Choice of home becomes particularly important in such cases and families and friends may have a particular role to play in advising staff and supporting the person.

ETHNIC MINORITY AND IMMIGRANT GROUPS AND RESIDENTIAL CARE

Research shows that minority ethnic groups are under-represented in care homes for people with dementia, implying that many families from these groups are caring for people in the later phases of dementia at home. There are likely to be a number of reasons for this. First, some ethnic groups have strong cultural values regarding looking after older family members within the family. Second, there may be stigma in some ethnic groups regarding dementia, and some families may feel ashamed if a member goes to live in a care home. Finally and probably most importantly, ethnic minority families may (with some reason) feel that care homes that cater largely for the majority population may not offer culturally sensitive care to minorities. Suitable arrangements may not be made for food preferences, personal care, language issues and religious observance. There are no easy answers to this. Numbers of older people with dementia from minority ethnic groups are currently small and there are few care homes that cater specifically for particular ethnic groups. As in other aspects of their lives, those from minority ethnic groups who have dementia may face a harder battle to get their needs met in a society very different from their own.

GAY, LESBIAN, BISEXUAL AND TRANS-GENDERED PEOPLE WITH DEMENTIA AND RESIDENTIAL CARE

As we mentioned in Chapter 1, the issues of care and support for gay, lesbian, bisexual and trans-gendered (GLBT) people with dementia are the same as for others, but factors in their situation may create challenges if the person enters residential care. Sadly, some GLBT people become estranged from their families and may enter residential care because of lack of support in the community. If the person has been living with and supported by a same-sex partner, that person will of course want to continue to visit and support the person. In theory there should not be an issue with this: the principles of relationship-based care should apply in all cases and the person's partner should be welcomed by care home staff just as other family members and friends would be. In practice, attitudes can sometimes create barriers. Sadly, some care home staff may express negative attitudes towards GLBT people. Also, some couples may be reluctant to 'come out' to care home staff, either because they have always kept the nature of their relationship to themselves or through fear of possible negative reactions. Partnership with care home staff will be enhanced by a clear shared understanding of the nature of the relationship between a resident and the person who regularly visits and provides support. Sometimes an open discussion with the home manager at the point of choosing a care home can facilitate that understanding, to the benefit of all concerned.

BEHAVIOUR THAT CARE HOME STAFF FIND DIFFICULT

Just as families and friends may find some aspects of the behaviours of a person with dementia difficult, so do care home staff. When the person appears to be distressed or agitated, when they become aggressive or persist in wanting to get away from the home, staff can feel as stressed and burdened as family members do. The strategies that staff can use to respond to such behaviour are the same as those set out in Chapter 5 and should embrace an individualised approach based on knowing the person and their life history. Family members and friends can obviously contribute by telling staff about the person's life and suggesting strategies that they have used in the past. Understanding about the person's routines can help in adapting care: did they used to get up early for work, did they do night shifts or did they regularly pick children up from school at a certain time? Also knowing about previous roles and activities can help staff to understand behaviour – did they like to be outdoors, were they in positions of authority in their work, did they do manual labour?

Other difficulties can arise from the fact that the person is now living in a communal environment. Arguments may occur between residents if they lack sufficient space or are not supported adequately by staff. An issue that can sometimes arise is that of sexual relationships developing between residents. People with moderate dementia can sometimes demonstrate sexual behaviour towards others without being aware of the implications. This can be challenging and needs to be responded to very carefully and sensitively. The onset of old age or a cognitive impairment does not take away the need for affection, intimacy or relationships, and care homes should have approaches that recognise this but also protect the person as potentially vulnerable.

Research suggests that some care home staff may resort to sedating medication as their main response to behaviour they find difficult, rather than looking for more person-centred solutions. This is despite the considerable drawbacks of such medication discussed in Chapter 5, not least of which is that it rarely works. Family members and friends should ask the manager of a home at initial visit how they respond to distressed or agitated behaviour and what their attitude and approach is to the use of sedating medication.

Concerns about standards of care

Family members and friends visiting a person may be critical of aspects of the care the person is receiving. Broadly speaking, such criticisms can arise for three main reasons.

FAMILY MEMBERS AND FRIENDS BELIEVING THAT
CARE IS NOT UP TO THEIR OWN STANDARDS

Many family carers provide a very high standard of care, particularly in terms of helping a person keep clean, fed and well presented. They may feel that the care home staff are not keeping up the standards that they would want or would provide themselves. They may feel that the person is dressed untidily, is not clean, or they may perceive that the person is losing weight. It is perhaps inevitable that hard-pressed care staff, who have to provide for many residents, may not be able to do things as well as a family member devoting their whole time to one person. At the same time, it is possible that standards are not as they should be at the home. This could be the result of staff shortages, poorly trained staff or an ethos of corner-cutting. A good relationship with the home or unit manager will help families and friends understand the home and its circumstances, and make them feel that they can speak up if they sense that standards are slipping. Dialogue with the manager may also lead to family members assisting as appropriate with caring activities such as supervising mealtimes.

DIFFERENCES OF OPINION REGARDING
THE MOST APPROPRIATE CARE

Sometimes the issue that family members and friends have is not that the home is giving poor care, but that aspects of care are not as they would want it, or, in their view, not what the person with dementia would want if they could express a choice. Perhaps the person's hair has been done differently; they are eating (and apparently enjoying) food that they would not normally eat; or taking part in activities that they would not normally consider. Maybe the staff are responding to aspects of the person's behaviour in ways that family members do not regard as appropriate. In some cases family members and friends need to act as advocates for the person and inform staff of their preferences – for example, if a life-long vegetarian was eating meat, or the person was doing things that were against their long-held religious principles. In other cases it may be more appropriate to take a more open-minded and tolerant view. One situation that might arise is that the care home staff use toys or dolls as means of promoting activity (see Chapter 4). Family members may be shocked that their relative is playing with children's toys but, as we have discussed, such activities may be appropriate for the person's abilities and may well enhance well-being. Discussion with staff about the rationale for certain activities may help relieve family members' reservations about some aspects of dementia care that might appear inappropriate but which actually reflect good practice.

CONCERNS ABOUT ABUSIVE, NEGLECTFUL OR EXPLOITATIVE PRACTICES

Sadly, as we discussed in Chapter 5, people with dementia are vulnerable to abuse, neglect and exploitation, and care home staff may in rare cases carry out such acts. If family members or friends suspect (or witness) that a member of staff is in some way abusing any resident, they should tell the manager at once and, if no action appears to be taken, contact the appropriate local government department, regulator or police.

> 'We knew things weren't perfect in the home, but what was the alternative? To take Mum to another place that would probably have the same sort of problems. We were between the devil and the deep blue sea as we knew this home was the best for Dad as he could still keep contact with her. There was always family visiting her and we felt that that might offer some protection.'

> 'If you do make a critical comment in the care home you can end up being treated as an "interfering relative". Families mustn't be afraid to speak up because they think it could have repercussions on the care of their loved ones. If they don't, nothing will change.'

Conclusion: care homes are places to live!

We would not wish to end this chapter on such a negative note. Care homes, along with dementia care overall have come a very long way since the days of Morecambe and Wise! There are many good care homes providing comfortable, pleasant and stimulating places for people with dementia to live. Family members and friends can be assured that their loved ones are being looked after well and can help enhance the person's well-being by staying involved and supporting the care home's staff.

CHAPTER 7

Completing the Journey

The Phase of Advanced Dementia

The characteristics of advanced dementia

The latter phase of dementia is known as 'advanced' or 'severe' dementia. In this phase a person's cognitive difficulties become profound and are commonly accompanied by increasing physical frailty. We have pointed out previously that dementia is a terminal condition and advanced dementia leads to a person's death, although some people can stay in this phase for some time. The goals of care in advanced dementia are the same as in all phases of the condition – that a person has as good a quality of life as possible and experiences well-being. In achieving these goals, however, those caring for the person will need to focus on physical care to a greater extent than previously. Family members or friends may be undertaking that caring role, or they may be supporting the person in a residential care setting. Either way, they will need to come to terms with the final change in their relationship with the person, because the progression of dementia can cause a person to lose the ability to communicate with or even to recognise their loved ones. They will also need to prepare for the person's eventual death.

As with the shift from early to moderate dementia, it is not possible to precisely draw a line between moderate and advanced dementia, or to say how long these phases will last. In advanced dementia, the difficulties encountered during the moderate phase progress, resulting in a person becoming totally dependent and retaining little awareness of their surroundings.

Advanced dementia usually involves the following:

- A person's ability to communicate verbally becomes progressively lessened. As well as having difficulties expressing themselves, they may appear not to understand words (known as 'receptive aphasia'). Their verbal communications may consist of repeated words, phrases or utterances that are difficult to understand. Alternatively they may be completely non-verbal and just communicate with noises, facial expressions or movements.

- Disorientation becomes increasingly marked. A person may have great difficulty in recognising where they are or where other places are. They may have limited conception of time. Most significantly, they may also lose the ability to recognise other people, including close friends and family members and even their partner or children. When shown themselves in a mirror or photograph, it is possible they will not recognise themselves.

- Memory loss and cognitive decline also become profound and a person is likely to be able to carry out only very simple activities. Their field of attention becomes reduced and they often do not appear to notice what is happening around them. Their behaviour becomes limited and often repetitive. A consequence of this is that behaviour that others find difficult, such as restless or agitated behaviour, tends to lessen.

- A person is likely to need complete help with activities of daily living including washing, dressing and eating.

- A person gradually loses control of their bladder and bowel functions and can become incontinent of urine and faeces.

- A person is likely to become increasingly physically frail and may lose the ability to walk unaided.

Faced with such decline, family members and friends may feel estranged from a person, especially if they are living in a care home, and may reduce visits. Those directly caring for the person may struggle to find the motivation to do so because of the physical demands and uncertainty of what difference they are making. These are pertinent issues, but in this chapter we will try to show that people in the advanced phase of dementia can have a good quality of life and experience well-being, and families and friends can help them do so.

> 'My husband had become very acquiescent. He could just about walk about, he had lost much of his speech and he wasn't aggressive towards me. I thought, "I can cope for six months."'

Well-being and ill-being in advanced dementia

When carrying out training sessions with nurses and care staff, we often ask participants to undertake a little 'thought experiment'. We would encourage readers to try it as well. Sit back comfortably in your chair and shut your eyes. Then try to imagine you had woken up this morning and could not remember anything at all. Think of yourself lying in bed, with absolutely no memory of anything that had happened before. Try to imagine what your thoughts and feelings would be if you found yourself in this situation.

What were your reactions to this exercise? Those taking part in our training sessions often suggest that they would experience emotions such as anxiety, fear or frustration, and their thoughts would be along the lines of 'What has happened to me?', 'Where am I?' or 'What should I do now?' (Some, more mischievously, remark that it would depend on who they woke up next to!)

These responses are possible, but they imply that the person retains some residual memory of the time before they woke up. To feel anxious, fearful or frustrated in this situation, one needs to have some sense of things having changed for the worse – an awareness that one used to have a memory and that there are things that one has forgotten. As we have seen in Chapter 3, people in the early phase of dementia sometimes experience these feelings because of their awareness that their memory is becoming unreliable. In this chapter, however, we are considering advanced dementia, when the person's memory difficulties have become so profound that they may not remember *anything* – they may have no conception of any time prior to the moment of their waking.

Try to put yourself in this situation and carry out the exercise again. This time, consider what would influence the way you felt if you woke up remembering absolutely nothing.

Participants in our training sessions have responded that their feelings in this case would not necessarily be negative ones. Many have recognised that it would be likely to depend on physical factors – when they woke up were they cold or hot, comfortable or stiff? Did they wake up to a quiet and pleasant environment or to lots of noise and glaring light? Importantly, in what circumstances did they wake up? Did they wake naturally, in their own time? Or were they woken by someone roughly pulling their bedclothes off, manhandling them, making loud, harsh, incomprehensible noises and pulling them out of their nice warm comfortable beds?

In short, a person's reactions in this situation will be a function of how they experience their surroundings through their basic senses. Their feelings will be either positive or negative depending upon their level of comfort: how pleasant or otherwise their environment is and how other people interact with them. If all these factors are positive the person will experience well-being, and if they are negative the person will experience ill-being. This is the world of someone with advanced dementia. It is a world where the person interacts with their surroundings at the sensory-motor level – experiencing the world through the fundamental senses of sight, hearing, smell, taste and touch, and responding with basic 'motor activity'. But the person still has the capacity to have good or bad feelings and their feelings are going to depend on those around them. If those caring for them can create an environment that is warm, comfortable, secure, free from stressors and with meaningful human contact, well-being will result.

Relationships with a person with advanced dementia

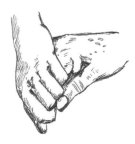

How can we communicate meaningfully with someone who apparently does not understand language and who cannot respond to what is being said to them? How can we have any kind of relationship with a person who does not seem to know who we are, even if we are their closest family or lifelong partner? When the person reaches the phase of advanced dementia, the contrast between their present state and the way they once were is at its most extreme and the tendency for family members and friends to feel that 'it isn't really him/her' and to shy away from the person is understandably at its greatest. We may even feel that the person has been 'lost' leaving a body that still functions up to a point but with those things that make up a human being broken down by the relentless onset of neurological disease. Those who have come to think in this way may have given up the struggle to maintain a relationship with their family member.

We assume from the fact that you are still reading this book that you are not among those families, though you may well not blame them for feeling this way. Maintaining a relationship with a person with advanced dementia requires faith that one is doing the right thing and that at some level the person knows that one is there. For many, of course, this is not a problem. The person with dementia is their spouse, partner, mother or father, and they will be there for the person come what may. But for all who give their time to someone with advanced dementia, the question, 'Am I making a difference?' is a pertinent one.

> 'Dad loved Mum just as much as he'd always loved her, I know that. When she was in the late stages I can remember him saying, "You'll always be my flower." He'd stroke her and say "it was for better or for worse" and things like that. He never said it was too much.'

One way of answering this question is to recognise that small successes have enhanced significance. It can be the case that, with the right environment and care, abilities and functions assumed to be lost can return, albeit temporarily. At these times we see a window into the person who was.

> 'When I brought my husband home and we went through the door, my husband saw the picture on the wall that he'd painted. He gave me a big smile and said "Home"; he hadn't said an intelligible word for months.'

Communication in advanced dementia

Communication at this stage of dementia is just as important for a person, if not more so, because of their reduced ability to interact with the world. If communication through language is not possible with a person with advanced dementia, then other modes of interaction must be used. Para-verbal and non-verbal communication are technical-sounding terms for simple concepts. 'Para-verbal' refers to the strategies we use to add feeling or emotion to what we say. It includes such things as our tone of voice, the speed and volume of our speech, the facial expressions that accompany our speech and the other actions or gestures we use. All these things both reflect our emotions and convey our emotions to others – sometimes whether we want them to or not!

Through para-verbal means we may convey feelings of happiness, sadness, anger, love, fear, boredom, reassurance and so on.

The relevance of this for interacting with a person with advanced dementia is that many who work with this group of people believe that their ability to recognise para-verbal aspects of communication may still be present after their ability to understand language has been lost and their sense of well- or ill-being may be influenced by how we speak to them. Recall our thought experiment earlier in this chapter, when we asked you to imagine waking up with no memory. Compare how you would feel if the first person you came across after you woke up had an angry expression and spoke to you in a harsh, loud, unfriendly tone, with your feelings if they had a friendly smile and spoke softly but clearly, in a warm and reassuring manner. Your sense of well-being is more likely to be enhanced in the latter case than the former.

This of course implies that we actually talk to people with advanced dementia. Although we may feel that talking to them is pointless because they will not understand what we are saying, we should continue to do so. In the first place, we do not know for sure that they cannot understand: it is possible that they can, even when their ability to respond has been lost. Second, speech is such an integral part of human relationships that a completely silent relationship (unless one is deaf) does not seem right and we may surmise that a person with dementia would at some level expect a person interacting with them to speak to them. Finally, as we have seen, there is the possibility of the person perceiving and maybe responding to the feelings that we convey para-verbally while speaking to them – without speech those feelings cannot be properly expressed.

> 'I don't think my wife recognises anyone now although I do think she sometimes recognises my voice but I am not sure she registers who I am.'

The other way we can communicate with a person with advanced dementia is non-verbally. People with advanced dementia have very limited fields of attention and are likely to only be able to attend visually to people or things that are close to and in front of them. Family members and friends will need to be aware of this and, applying the principles of dementia empathy, use aspects of non-verbal communication to maximise the possibility of the person being able to attend to them. Sitting straight and looking directly at the person and sitting close to the person and in front of them will help them focus, attend and – perhaps – recognise who is there.

Touch may also be a good way of maintaining a relationship with a person with advanced dementia. Often a person seems to respond more to touch than to visual cues or voices. How touch is used will depend on the nature of the previous relationship and what the parties involved have been used to, but often simply holding the person's hand is an effective way of communicating that one is there for them.

> 'Even though my husband couldn't talk back, we could talk to him. Nothing got in the way to alarm him; he could put all his energies into just living, and I think he was content.'

Activity and advanced dementia

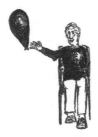

It is tempting to take the view that for people with advanced dementia activity is impossible, or at least unnecessary. We may feel that a person's communication difficulties, memory loss and restricted field of attention will lead to their being unable to participate in activities in any meaningful sense of the word. It is certainly true that by the phase of advanced dementia many of the social and diversional activities we discussed in Chapter 4 would be beyond the abilities or comprehension of the person. This does not mean, however, that people with advanced dementia have no need of activity or that there are no activities that are suitable for them. Many people with advanced dementia show signs of wanting to be active and appear to appreciate it when others help them with activities.

Because cognitive and language difficulties are so profound in advanced dementia, the best activities for such people are those that 'bypass' intellectual processes, operate at the level of the person's primary senses and involve basic actions – what we like to call 'sensory-motor activities'. Some examples from our own nursing experience may serve to illustrate the range of possibilities:

- Carol was unsteady on her feet but could walk about with someone to support her. She had lost the use of language and apparently had little awareness of her surroundings. However, when a feather duster was put in her hand she became much more animated. She went about the room poking her feather duster into corners and across surfaces to clean them and continued with this activity as long as staff were able to help her.

- Bessie had also lost the use of language and could not stand unaided. She had a reputation for grumpiness. One day a music session was taking place. A nurse offered her a triangle, but Bessie did not understand what it was for. The nurse then held the triangle up by its string and gave Bessie the sounding rod. After a while Bessie got the hang of making a noise by hitting the triangle with the rod, which she proceeded to do continuously. She evidently enjoyed this activity because her face went into the biggest smile the nurses had ever seen from her.

- Henry had always enjoyed sports but was now chair-bound. Nurses tried to engage him in games of 'catch' with a soft ball but he did not understand the concept of the game. He did, however, enjoy hitting back a balloon that was floated towards him; this simpler activity was understandable to him and engaged his interest.

- Angela was also chair-bound and often appeared tense, sometimes crying out unintelligibly. A staff member who had an interest in complementary medicine carried out a simple hand massage with Angela, using lavender oil. Angela appeared to attend to this activity and for a while afterwards she seemed a bit more relaxed and less inclined to call out.

- Stan had been a dog-lover all his life but was now unable to speak or walk. His family bought him a life-sized soft-toy dog that lay on his lap and Stan enjoyed stroking and playing with it.

- Eve often waved her hands about and tried to reach out for things. She liked a fibre-optic electric lamp that had a spray of illuminated fibres that waved about and changed colour. She enjoyed stroking the fibres, making them move about and looking at the resulting light effects.

We could offer many more examples, but the stories we have related here will perhaps serve to illustrate some basic points about activity with people with advanced dementia:

- Activity is possible with most people with advanced dementia. All but the most disabled will retain some awareness of their surroundings and want to remain engaged.

- The examples of activity that we have described are linked by their simplicity. All avoid the need for complex cognitive processing and involve basic sensory stimulation or motor actions.

- The gains from such activities are small ones and a person may only be able to concentrate for a short period of time. However, while taking part in the activity, the person appears to show enjoyment. Family members and friends should value such small gains – even brief and simple activities are better than no activity.

Helping people with advanced dementia with activities of daily living

By the phase of advanced dementia, a person is likely to be totally dependent on others for carrying our activities of daily living such as personal care (washing, dressing and meeting continence needs) and eating and drinking. If the person is living in a residential care setting, this help will be provided by care staff but, as we discussed in Chapter 6, family members and friends may still sometimes offer assistance, especially at mealtimes. If the person is living at home, care staff may come to the house to carry out particular activities such as getting the person bathed and dressed. In some circumstances, however, family carers may need to develop the skills of helping the person with activities of daily living.

PERSONAL CARE

Washing and dressing a person with advanced dementia are intimate tasks and family carers may well feel uncomfortable undertaking them. By this phase, the person may not be able to offer any assistance and so the activity must be supported by others. The person may have lost awareness of their need to go to the toilet or, if they are aware, be unable to meet their continence needs themselves or communicate those needs to others.

Giving personal care, including continence care, as well as being embarrassing, can be time-consuming and tiring at the best of times. This is when a person co-operates with, or at least does not resist, what is being done. Sometimes, however, the person will resist care that is in their best interest. Broadly speaking, there are two reasons for this, both of which can be appreciated by recalling our 'thought experiment' at the beginning of the chapter. First, by this phase of their condition, the person has effectively no memory and their cognitive processes are considerably impaired, so they have little or no conception of what is being done to them, or why. They are aware, however, that others are doing things to their body that they do not understand, and they may well find them uncomfortable and feel threatened by them. In those circumstances, resistance is perhaps a natural reaction.

The second reason for resistance is related to the first and stems from the way that those giving personal care go about the activity. Remember that in our thought experiment we asked you to consider how a person with no memory might feel if they were woken by someone roughly pulling their bedclothes off, manhandling them, making loud, harsh, incomprehensible noises and pulling them out of their nice warm comfortable beds. Sadly, some care staff (and perhaps some family carers) fail to realise that their personal manner is likely to be perceived by the person, who will react resistively if they are approached in the wrong way.

It follows from this discussion that those giving personal care will minimise ill-being in the person, reduce resistance and thereby make the experience of giving personal care a more pleasant one for both the person and themselves if they follow some basic principles:

- Make sure you are well prepared – get everything you need in advance and keep everything to hand. The person may become more disorientated and agitated if you have to keep breaking off the activity to find things.

- Use good communication principles throughout (see earlier). Make sure the person knows you are there before beginning the activity. Talk to them about what you are going to do in a calm and pleasant voice – they may understand what you are saying or at least be reassured by your tone of voice. Show them the things you are using (clothes, toiletries, etc.) – they may recognise them.

- Consider using background music as a pleasant distraction to the task in hand.

- Sometimes the person can help a little; encourage them to do so if possible.

- If the person continues to resist, it can sometimes be helpful to leave them for a while and return later. Always try to keep your temper – as we have seen, the person may well perceive negative emotions and may respond with still greater resistance.

- If resistance is persistent, or the person responds aggressively despite these approaches, and the activity has to be done, plan how to carry it out in as safe and dignified a way as possible. As a last resort, a degree of restraint of the person may be necessary and, if this is the case, then more than one helper will be needed to prevent injury to the person or others. Any restraint used should be the minimum needed to get the task completed.

NUTRITION AND ADVANCED DEMENTIA

We discussed nutrition, eating and drinking at some length in Chapter 5 and the principles examined in that chapter apply in the same way in the advanced phase of dementia. In this phase, however, a person's progressive cognitive and physical difficulties can lead to extra challenges for those caring for them. First, the person may lose the ability to feed themselves, even after trying strategies such as finger foods, and will need to be fed by others. As we have discussed, in care homes or hospitals, responsibility for ensuring adequate nutrition lies with the nursing and care staff, but family members and friends may want to assist at mealtimes. Sometimes feeding a person with advanced dementia is easy, because the person appears to relish their food and readily opens their mouth and swallows. In other cases, more skill and patience are required. Principles of successfully feeding a person with dementia include the following.

- Ensure the person is awake and alert.

- Ensure the person is as upright as possible.

- Orientate the person as far as possible, by telling them what you are doing or showing them the plate and cutlery.

- If the person doesn't open their mouth, don't assume they don't want to eat. Find a way of assisting them to recognise that you are offering them food. Sometimes gently putting a spoon to their lips with a little food on it will encourage them to open their mouth.

- Take your time. Don't rush the person or try to give them too big pieces of food, even if they seem to want them. You may risk the person choking or aspirating (see later).

- Make mealtimes pleasant. People with advanced dementia like eating and drinking as much as the rest of us, and a pleasant relaxed mealtime will enhance their well-being. Again, gentle background music can enhance the experience of eating. Use the opportunity for interaction, or at least being with the person in a companionable way.

Swallowing problems

There are risk areas when helping a person with advanced dementia to eat. 'Dysphagia' is the term used to describe difficulty with swallowing. A possible consequence of dysphagia is 'aspiration', which occurs when food goes from the mouth into the person's windpipe rather than their oesophagus. In severe cases, the windpipe can become blocked, leading to choking, and persistent episodes of aspiration can lead to chest infections, including aspiration pneumonia, which is sometimes a cause of death among people with advanced dementia. Dysphagia can result from a number of causes, including a person over-filling their mouth, swallowing without chewing, prolonged chewing or holding food in the mouth. Occasionally the person's swallowing reflex becomes impaired.

A person should be watched carefully when eating for signs of dysphagia and aspiration, which should be suspected if the person persistently coughs or makes a gurgling noise after swallowing. Risks can be minimised if time is taken with meals and the person does not take in large mouthfuls. In some cases, thickening fluids and a soft, fork-mashable or smooth diet may be needed, but pureed food should not be given simply as an easy option.

Another solution that is sometimes considered is for a person to receive artificial feeding, sometimes known as tube feeding, with food being passed down a tube directly into the person's stomach. Sometimes the tube is threaded down to the stomach via the nose (nasal-gastric feeding) or, more commonly in dementia care, the tube is surgically passed through the person's skin into the stomach (percutaneous endoscopic gastronomy or 'PEG' feeding). This is a controversial and emotive issue because severe dysphagia is often a sign that the person is nearing the end of their life and we may question whether the attempt to prolong life through artificial feeding is justified. We will consider this further in the next chapter.

RESPONDING TO INCONTINENCE

In advanced dementia, a person may become 'doubly incontinent', meaning that they have lost all control over their bladder and bowel functions, though good practice in helping the person meet their continence needs in the earlier stages may delay the onset of incontinence (see Chapter 5). Once a person has lost control over their bladder and/or bowels, an assessment about the use of incontinence pads should be carried out. While the person is still mobile, the use of elasticated pull-up pads may be the best option to help promote their dignity and encourage independence. Later, when the person is immobile, it is essential that incontinence pads are absorbent enough and fit well. No-one should be left for long periods in incontinence pads and if they become soiled they should be changed as soon as possible both discreetly and sensitively.

While it may be tempting to consider the use of a catheter for people who become incontinent of urine, this is not recommended for people in the advanced stage of dementia unless there is an urgent medical need, such as acute urine retention. Catheters can be a source of significant discomfort and distress and there is an increased risk of urinary tract infections if they are left in place for any length of time.

MANAGING PAIN AND DISCOMFORT

As discussed in Chapter 5, pain can be a significant cause of distress. Research has shown that pain in dementia often goes unrecognised. Consider that someone in the advanced phase may have limited mobility or movement and may be in one position for a long time. They may have pain from other physical conditions. In addition, they have reduced ability to communicate their pain or discomfort. It is therefore essential that we observe for signs of pain using non-verbal means. There are some specific assessment tools that have been designed for clinicians to help them recognise and treat pain in dementia. Their basic principle is to observe for gestures, facial expressions and noises that might indicate pain or distress especially on movement and when providing personal care. If you notice any of these symptoms, then do consider pain relief and seek advice.

The main principles of providing comfort in the phase of advanced dementia include the following.

- Ensure the person is pain free by observing their behaviour and giving adequate pain relief.

- Maintain comfort through pressure-relieving mattresses and gentle repositioning.

- Keep skin clean and dry by gentle washing, drying and use of moisturising skin creams.

- Use well-fitting continence pads and make regular changes.

- Keep the mouth moist and clean.

- Use aromatherapy (for example, lavender and lemon balm oil or familiar perfumes and air fresheners).

- Play familiar, soothing music or sing favourite songs.

- Talk to the person while giving care.

- Have low lighting.

- Have soft textures for the person to hold and touch such as soft material or toys.

- Use touch, including gentle hand massage, stroking someone's face, holding them.

- Be with the person and let them know you are there.

Approaching the end of life

The profound cognitive difficulties of the phase of advanced dementia, along with increased physical frailty, characterised by progressive issues with mobility, eating and drinking, signify that a person's life is drawing to a close. As with other phases of dementia, it is hard to put a timescale on how long the phase of advanced dementia will last – for some, death may come within weeks or months while others may live on for some years. Death is always possible at any time, however, and sooner or later it will become clear that the person will not live much longer. Those caring for them will need to make decisions about how they should be looked after to try to ensure a peaceful death. In the next chapter we will consider care for people with dementia at the end of their life, the role of family members and friends in care and treatment decisions, and also their own needs for understanding and support during this time.

> 'Having visited the home for two years I have seen other people go downhill and die. I think I have reconciled myself to the fact that my wife is maybe entering that process; that she will die, but who knows how long that will take? Six months, two years, but I don't really want to know.'

CHAPTER 8

The End of Life

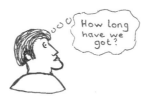

As we have discussed, dementia is sadly an incurable, progressive and terminal condition. This means that all those who develop dementia will die with the condition – it is estimated that one in three people over the age of 65 will die with dementia (Knapp and Prince 2007). It is not necessarily the case, however, that all will die *of* dementia, and not all will reach the phase of advanced dementia before they die. But dementia as a cause of death is often underestimated and as a consequence the opportunity to provide good end of life care may be missed. In this chapter we will consider end of life care whenever it occurs during the journey through dementia, and wherever it occurs – people with dementia may die in a care home or in their own home, or in hospital. The end of life may be a time of decision making and we will discuss the role of family members and friends in those decisions, given that the person with dementia may not be able to contribute themselves. We will also consider how family members and friends can support the person in achieving a peaceful death and how they can meet their own needs for information, support and comfort at this time. (We will not here address the vexed topic of assisted suicide, as this has been covered in Chapter 3. We will also not provide a comprehensive account of all aspects of end of life care, only those aspects where dementia may create particular issues.)

What is meant by 'end of life'?

For the purpose of this chapter we will consider end of life in relation to the generally quite short period when it is clear that a person's physical condition, regardless of their phase of dementia, has deteriorated to the point where death is imminent and likely to occur within a few weeks or days. This stage is accompanied with symptoms such as:

- deterioration in swallowing

- loss of weight

- reduction in awareness

- reduction in peripheral circulation

- altered respiration pattern.

As some of these are similar to symptoms of advanced dementia, the exact end of life stage for a person in this phase of dementia can be difficult to detect. As a result, this stage of advanced dementia is sometimes described as 'dwindling'. It is during this time that the most significant decisions need to be reached and when the person, their family and friends need particular care and support.

At the same time, we must also acknowledge that in cases of sudden death – for example, from a heart attack, stroke or accident – there is often no time for a person to experience end of life care. In such cases our attention must be with family members and friends, for whom coming to terms with the person's death can be compromised by the lack of opportunity to prepare for it.

What causes death among people with dementia?

As suggested earlier, death can occur at any phase during the progression of dementia. This is of course because the majority of people with dementia are older people, with dementia being most prevalent in the oldest age groups. Some people will have developed long-term age-related conditions such as cardio-vascular and respiratory diseases or cancer prior to developing dementia (as we have seen, a history of cardio-vascular disease increases the risk of dementia), or may acquire such conditions after the onset of dementia. Many people die *with* dementia rather than dying *of* dementia. Some will only be in the early phase of dementia and may be able to take part in end of life decision making and care planning. In practice, only a minority of people live through to the advanced phase. As mentioned, sudden death is possible, from a range of causes.

If the person does reach the phase of advanced dementia, they may die of a condition related to that phase. As mentioned in Chapter 7, people with advanced dementia are often immobile or bed bound and at increased risk of swallowing difficulties in which aspiration can lead to a severe and often fatal chest infection. In addition, people's immune systems are often compromised leaving them more at risk from pneumonia, urinary or other infections and less responsive to antibiotics. Vascular conditions such as blood clotting may also be exacerbated by immobility. Sometimes a person simply seems to 'fade away' and dementia itself may be recorded as the cause of death.

> 'He recovered from a number of chest infections, with or without antibiotics. On numerous occasions, when the GP came to visit he would say that he might have a few days, even hours left and I would call all the family around. It was a roller-coaster of emotions every time.'

The feelings of family members and friends as end of life approaches

Perhaps inevitably, family members and friends have mixed feelings as they become aware that a person is nearing the end of their life. Sadness and grief at the impending loss is often tempered by a measure of relief that the person's journey through dementia is coming to a conclusion. Some will for some time have been mourning the loss of the person as they once were – it is recognised that family members and friends can begin to go through a grieving process as dementia is identified and will increasingly feel bereaved as the condition progresses and the person loses more and more of their previous nature and abilities. Some will have more or less come to terms with the person's death when the time comes and may regard it as a 'release', both for the person with dementia and for themselves.

> 'I used to pray that my mum would die sooner than she did die. When Mum did die I obviously cried but not for my mum being dead, I was just relieved.'

> 'There can be an initial sense of relief and release because the person has become very disabled and you are relieved they are at peace.'

Many others, however, will remain devoted to the person and will feel the pain of pending loss and bereavement regardless of how long the person has had dementia or how far it has progressed. Such feelings may be particularly acute if the person has young-onset dementia and is dying at a relatively early age, but grief is of course not age related. Family members and friends must be sensitive to each others' feelings. Saying to a grieving spouse that 'it's for the best' will be of no comfort if the couple have been devoted to each other and the person left behind is devastated at their loss.

How would we want to die?

This may seem to some to be a rather blunt and intrusive question. Death is an uncomfortable subject to many from Western cultures and speaking about death (or even thinking about it) is still often regarded as taboo. However, reflecting upon how we ourselves would like to die will help us understand the issues faced by a person with dementia as they near the end of life and how to assist them to have the death that they would want.

Broadly speaking, we would imagine that most people would want their death to include these principles:

- We would want to be told the truth about what is happening to us, so we can prepare ourselves and say goodbye to family and friends. We would want to be aware of our medical status and the intended medical and nursing plan of care. We would want to know if attempts would be made to resuscitate us if our heart or breathing stopped.

- We would want to die in a place of our choosing. For many of us, this would be our home, but some who are living alone or do not want their families to have to care for them might prefer to die in a setting where professionals are available to give care.

- We would want to be as physically comfortable and free of pain as possible. If we were unable to meet our own daily living needs, we would want these to be done for us in a way that maintained comfort and dignity.

- We would want the option of not prolonging our life if it was clear that the end was imminent. We would want to be aware of any medical treatments and procedures that doctors or nurses intended to do to us and to be able to refuse any treatments that we did not wish to receive.

- If we had a faith, we would want to be able to carry out religious or spiritual activities (or have them done for us) and our body to be treated according to our religious beliefs after our death.

- We would not want to die alone. Ideally we would want to be with loved ones when we died, but if that was not possible we would want to have people with us who had our interests at heart and could offer comfort and support.

- If we became unconscious or unaware as death approached, we would want to know that we were still being watched over and treated with dignity and compassion.

- We would want our loved ones to be supported, looked after and comforted, both in the time leading up to our death and following it.

It is sadly the case that many people who do not have dementia experience deaths that fail to meet many of these principles. If this is the case, then what chances do people with dementia have of experiencing a 'good death'? In the next section we will discuss how dementia may compromise a person's experience at the end of life and how people with dementia may be helped to have as good an experience at this time as possible.

Dementia and end of life care

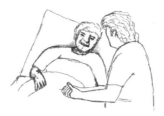

It will be apparent to readers that dementia is likely to compromise a person experiencing a death that meets the principles set out earlier. Depending on how far they are through the dementia journey (as well as their physical state as end of life approaches) the person is likely to have difficulties with communication, awareness and decision making and all will affect their experience. We will consider each aspect and how family members and friends may help the person at this time.

COMMUNICATION DIFFICULTIES

In the later phases of dementia, a person's language and communication difficulties will affect their ability to tell others how they are feeling or what their wishes are. They will also be unable to take in what others tell them about their condition. It can be particularly hard to tell if a person is experiencing pain or discomfort. Family members and friends may help by using their own knowledge of the person to try to judge their level of pain or discomfort. Signs of possible pain are increased confusion, agitation or restlessness, changes in sleep pattern, if the person appears more tense and rigid than usual or vocalises to a greater extent. It is particularly important when the person is being moved to observe for signs of distress that might indicate pain, such as grimacing, moaning, tears or protective body postures. Such changes should be reported to medical or nursing staff, who should respond by trying increased analgesia or other means of enhancing comfort.

As we discussed in Chapter 7, it is important that the person is still talked to as if they can understand what is being communicated to them. It is likely that they may comprehend at some level, and will feel reassured by family members' and friends' presence and continued willingness to interact with them.

AWARENESS

Are people with moderate or advanced dementia aware at this time that their life is coming to an end? In most cases it is impossible to answer this question and it is likely that we will assume that they have little or no awareness of what is happening to them. It may give us a degree of comfort to think this, because lack of awareness may mean less suffering for the person.

At the same time, if professionals such as doctors, nurses and care home staff – and family members and friends – believe that the person has no awareness of their situation, there may be negative consequences for them. At worst, it may lead to an attitude of 'it doesn't matter what we do, they won't know'. At least, the person's religious or spiritual preferences should be respected and gone through, even if they are not aware of any ritual or ceremony taking place. Also, they should continue to be treated with respect and dignity and their likely need for company supported. Family members and friends may need to advocate on behalf of the person with professional staff – or each other – if they feel that the person is not being treated with due respect or proper care is not being given.

DECISION MAKING

If a person lacks mental capacity at end of life, they will be prevented from taking part in decision making regarding their care and treatment and place of dying, and their wishes may not be known or acted upon. Research shows that the majority of people want to end their lives in familiar surroundings and most do not want to die in hospital. It is the case, however, that a large number of people in countries such as the UK do end their lives in hospital and people with dementia may be particularly likely to do so. This is sometimes because family carers feel unable to care for the person at home and sometimes that feeling is reinforced by professionals who may say that they lack the resources to provide proper nursing or medical support in the person's home. Care home staff may also believe that they lack the skills or resources to care for dying people and the person may be referred to hospital accordingly – although as we saw in Chapter 5 many hospital staff themselves may lack knowledge of dementia and skills of dementia care. Again, the person risks experiencing an undignified death. While hospital admission may be in the person's best interests in some cases, advocacy by family members and friends may in other cases allow the person to end their life in a more appropriate environment, cared for by people who know and respect them.

Treatment or care decisions that may need to be taken include whether to attempt to resuscitate the person if their heart or breathing stops; whether to use artificial feeding in cases of swallowing difficulties; and whether to give drugs or other treatments that might prolong the person's life. As we saw in Chapter 3, a person with dementia may make their preferences known while they still have capacity by drawing up an advance decision related to these areas and in most cases that decision would be legally binding, so long as it was properly drawn up and unambiguous. Alternatively, the person may, if legally possible in their country, appoint a family member or friend as their attorney, to make care decisions on their behalf. In the absence of such formal arrangements, family members and friends have no legal power to make decisions for the person, but good practice holds that doctors or nurses should consult family members when such decisions have to be made.

> 'During my husband's last chest infection, he looked weary; he couldn't hold up his head any more and his swallowing went completely. He was on a very low dose of oral antibiotics, and the doctor asked if I wanted to have him brought into hospital to have intravenous antibiotics and hydration, or if I wanted to keep him at home and let nature take its course.'

DO NOT ATTEMPT RESUSCITATION DECISIONS

In countries such as the UK, if the person is in hospital and a 'do not attempt resuscitation' (DNAR) decision has *not* been made, staff are obliged to attempt to resuscitate a person whose heart or breathing has stopped. Resuscitation can be undignified and uncomfortable for the person and is considered much less likely to be successful for people in later stages of dementia. Even if the person survives, they may experience further health problems and crisis situations before their eventual death.

DNAR decisions can only be taken by a doctor and family members or friends cannot direct doctors either to resuscitate the person or otherwise. The person themselves, through the medium of an advanced decision, can however express that they do not wish to be resuscitated in these circumstances and doctors should in most cases respect that wish.

At the same time it should not be the case that DNAR decisions are automatically made on all people with dementia who have serious illnesses. Resuscitation can prolong life and if the person is in the early phase of dementia they may experience many more good quality years if they recover from physical illness. We would oppose any health care system that discriminated against people with dementia by denying them treatment simply on the grounds that they had dementia – all such decisions should be taken in the best interests of the person, not the health care system.

ARTIFICIAL FEEDING

As discussed in Chapter 7, artificial feeding is sometimes proposed for people with advanced dementia who towards the end of life develop difficulties with swallowing. This is a highly controversial treatment in this context. While current advice does not suggest a blanket ban on artificial nutrition and hydration, neither naso-gastric tubes nor PEG feeding are recommended for the end of life. While it has been suggested that artificial feeding can improve the person's strength and abilities and can reduce pressure sores through enhancing the person's weight, there is no evidence that these benefits actually occur. In addition, introducing a nasal-gastric or PEG tube is uncomfortable and undignified for a person and leads to less contact with others through eating and drinking. Complications may arise if the tube becomes infected or dislodged, or if the person pulls it out. Although they may not take in much food orally, lack of desire to eat is common at the end of life and a person is likely to die of the underlying disease process rather than from starvation.

These seem to be powerful arguments against tube feeding and the procedure is nowadays rarely applied, but family members and friends may be consulted regarding its use. A person drawing up an advanced decision may wish to express their view regarding whether or not they would want artificial feeding if they had advanced dementia, or to advise a person acting as their legal attorney accordingly.

> 'I had to reassure the care team that now my husband could no longer swallow we would not be starving him to death because in the dying process he would feel neither hungry nor thirsty, provided his mouth was kept moist and clean.'

A good death?

Consider the following true story, as related by Michael, a care assistant in a nursing home:

> James had been resident in the home for about six months but he had become very disabled and completely dependent. He'd been an accountant by profession. His wife visited him a lot but he didn't seem to recognise her, he just mumbled to himself when she was there. Then he weakened markedly and it seemed clear that he would not live much longer. He was unable to eat solid food, and was fed through a feeding cup, though with difficulty. One afternoon at teatime, I brought James his drink and prepared to feed him. He looked at me intently and seemed to be trying to communicate with me. He said in a low, distinct voice, 'No…no…' I took the drink away without trying to feed him. That evening James died, peacefully, with his wife by his bedside.

What do we make of Michael's story? Do we believe that James was actually trying to communicate his real wish and what do we think of Michael's decision to go along with that apparent wish and take the drink away? Some writers have related anecdotal evidence of what have been termed 'intermittent spontaneous remissions': brief occasions, usually near to the end of life, when people with advanced dementia have had apparently lucid moments and have seemingly been able to communicate with others in a meaningful way. Was this one such moment? And if it was (or if it wasn't), did Michael do the right thing by not giving James the drink? It is highly unlikely that Michael hastened James's death by his decision and we may perhaps regard what he did as a humane individual act. Good care for people with dementia at the end of life is essentially the same as good care at every phase of the condition. The principles we have promoted throughout this book, of person-centredness, flexibility and treating people with dementia as individuals worthy of respect, apply as much at the end of life as at any other time in the person's journey through dementia.

'At the end we took positions of holding and cradling him and he just stopped with the rattling, strained noise and it eased off to normal breathing. The breaths got further and further apart, and he just slipped away – it was very peaceful.'

Support after death

The ability to provide comfort and well-being at the end of someone's life can be of particular concern because it is a memory many people are left with after the person has died. For those who are unable to achieve this because of circumstances out of their control, there can be an overriding sense of guilt and loss. In contrast, if we are able to ensure that a person has received the best care possible, then this can be replaced by feelings of satisfaction and reassurance.

After the person with dementia has died, family and friends continue to need support. The loss of a close relative or friend with dementia can have the same impact in terms of loss and bereavement as the death of anyone else even if it is anticipated and comes as a relief that the person is no longer 'suffering'. As with any death or loss, the practical arrangements for the funeral can keep people occupied initially and often during this time others are on hand to offer support and help. However, once this is over, there can be a gap left, especially for those who have been very involved in providing care whether at home or through regular visits to a care home. Some people have referred to 'delayed bereavement'. Family and friends should try to continue to support each other and bereavement counselling for those who are significantly affected may be a useful form of support.

'16 months after my husband died this bereavement shock hit me like a sledgehammer, and I didn't know what was happening to me, both physically and mentally; I still haven't really got it sorted yet.'

Conclusion

Suffering from Dementia or
Living with Dementia?

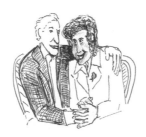

'So-and-so is suffering from dementia.' How often have we heard or read that phrase? We don't need to spell out its implications. The person is 'suffering'; they are experiencing anguish, ill-being and poor or non-existent quality of life and by extension their friends and families are too. Such phrases are part of the negative stereotype of dementia that the media still portrays. We occasionally read about well-known people or celebrities who have dementia and most likely they too will be described as 'suffering' from the condition.

But not all people with dementia are suffering, even well-known ones. Take, for example, the American pop singer and guitarist Glen Campbell. Early in 2011 he was diagnosed with Alzheimer's disease, at the age of 75, having experienced memory difficulties for some years. Instead of slipping out of the public eye to 'suffer' with his condition, Campbell embarked on a world concert tour, singing his famous songs 'Rhinestone Cowboy' and 'Wichita Linesman' to audiences of thousands and playing the guitar as well as he did in his youth. Look on Youtube and you will find excerpts from some of those concerts. What stands out from those clips is that, far from 'suffering', Campbell is having a whale of a time. He's making the best of the time he has left and is a classic example of someone *living with dementia*.

Another example is that of George Melly, the British jazz musician and singer who died in 2007 at the age of 80. George was diagnosed with vascular dementia yet continued to do live concerts until a few months before he died. With his wife Diana he made a film about vascular dementia and its impact on people with dementia and carers.

Of course, neither Glen Campbell nor George Melly could achieve these things unaided. The help and support received from family and friends were vital. In the case of Glen Campbell, three of his children played in his band, to support and guide him on stage, and his family were proactive in promoting his well-being. He used autocues to help him remember the song lyrics. George Melly was ably supported by his wife and by longstanding band members who were able to provide cues for familiar songs. With such assistance both performers' quality of life and sense of well-being were maximised – and they could continue to give fans pleasure as well.

We trust that our readers will recognise in these stories some of the themes and ideals of this book and that they will engender in them the hope that their own journey through dementia, for all its trials and difficulties, will not all be suffering. Family members and friends, with professional assistance, can make a big difference to the lives of people with dementia and, when the journey is over, they can have the satisfaction that they have helped the person to *live* with dementia.

References

Adelman, S., Blanchard, M., Rait, G., Leavey, G. and Livingston, G. (2011) 'Prevalence of dementia in African-Caribbean compared with UK-born White older people: two-stage cross-sectional study.' *British Journal of Psychiatry 199*, 2, 119–125.

Alzheimer's Association (2002) *African Americans and Alzheimer's Disease: The Silent Epidemic.* Available at www.alz.org/national/documents/report_africanamericanssilent epidemic.pdf, accessed on 20 April 2012.

Alzheimer's Association (2012) 'Alzheimer's Disease Facts and Figures.' *Alzheimer's and Dementia 8*, 2. Available at www.alz.org/downloads/Facts_Figures_2012.pdf, accessed on 20 April 2012.

Alzheimer's Society (2009) *Counting the Cost: Caring for People with Dementia on Hospital Wards.* London: Alzheimer's Society.

Alzheimer's Society (2011) *Optimising Treatment and Care for Behavioural and Psychological Symptoms of Dementia: A Best Practice Guide.* Available at: www.alzheimers.org.uk/bpsdguide, accessed on 2 August 2012.

Bayley, J. (1998) *Iris: A Memoir of Iris Murdoch.* London: Duckworth.

Graham, N. (2003) 'Editorial: Dementia and family care: the current international state of affairs.' *Dementia 2*, 147–149.

Kitwood, T. (1997) *Dementia Reconsidered: The Person Comes First.* Buckingham: Open University Press.

Knapp, M. and Prince, M. (eds) (2007) *Dementia UK – A Report into the Prevalence and Cost of Dementia.* London: Alzheimer's Society. Available at www.psige.org/psige-pdfs/Dementia_UK_Summary.pdf, accessed on 20 April 2012.

Leach, P. (1979) *Baby and Child.* London: Penguin.

Luengo-Fernandez, R., Leal, J. and Gray, A. (2010) *Dementia 2010: The Prevalence, Economic Cost and Research Funding of Dementia Compared with Other Major Diseases.* Cambridge: Alzheimer's Research Trust. Available at www.dementia2010.org/reports/Dementia2010Full.pdf, accessed on 20 April 2012.

Prince, M. and Jackson, J. (eds) (2009) *World Alzheimer Report 2009.* London: Alzheimer's Disease International. Available at www.alz.co.uk/research/files/WorldAlzheimerReport.pdf, accessed on 20 April 2012.

The Independent (2008) 'Brown calls for sensitivity over assisted suicide.' Available at www.independent.co.uk/news/uk/politics/brown-calls-for-sensitivity-over-assisted-suicide-1060787.html, accessed on 20 April 2012.

Thompson, R. and Heath, H. (2011) *Dignity in Dementia; Transforming General Hospital Care. Summary of Findings from Survey of Carers and People Living with Dementia.* London: Royal College of Nursing. Available at www.rcn.org.uk/__data/assets/pdf_file/0007/397564/RCN_Dementia_project_Summary_of_findings_from_carer_and_patient_survey_July_26_2011-11.pdf, accessed on 20 April 2012.

Resources for Families and Friends

Contact details for non-profit and government organisations in a selection of English-speaking countries that provide information about caring for people with dementia and offer support to family members and friends. Information is taken from the organisations' websites.

General

Alzheimer's Disease International – the global voice on dementia
Includes a list of worldwide dementia associations.
www.alz.co.uk/associations

United Kingdom

Age UK (formerly Age Concern and Help the Aged)
Provides information and advice for the elderly about benefits, care, age discrimination and computer courses.
0800 169 6565
www.ageuk.org.uk

Alzheimer Scotland
The leading dementia organisation in Scotland. Campaigns for the rights of people with dementia and their families, and provides an extensive range of innovative and personalised support services.
0808 808 3000
www.alzscot.org

Alzheimer's Society – leading the fight against dementia
0845 300 0336·
www.alzheimers.org.uk

Dementia – NHS Choices
Provides useful information about dementia, including causes, symptoms, diagnosis and treatment, with links to other useful resources.
www.nhs.uk/conditions/dementia

Dementia UK
Charity intent on improving the quality of life for people with dementia and their carers. It promotes and supports the development of Admiral Nurses, specialist nurses who support the needs of family carers and people with dementia. It has established 'Uniting Carers', a network of carers, and also provides training.
020 7874 7200
www.dementiauk.org

United States

Alzheimer's Association
The leading, global voluntary health organisation in Alzheimer's care and support, and the largest private, non-profit funder of Alzheimer's research. The Association works on a global, national and local level to enhance care and support for all those affected by Alzheimer's and related dementias.
24/7 helpline: 1-800-272-3900
www.alz.org

Alzheimer's Disease Education and Referral (ADEAR) Center
Founded in 1990 to 'compile, archive, and disseminate information concerning Alzheimer's disease' for health professionals, people with Alzheimer's disease and their families, and the public. The ADEAR Center is a service of the National Institute on Aging (NIA).
1-800-438-4380
www.nia.nih.gov/alzheimers

Eldercare Locator
A public service of the US Administration on Aging connecting to services for older adults and their families.
1-800-677-1116
www.eldercare.gov

Family Caregiver Alliance (FCA)
The first community-based non-profit organisation in the country to address the needs of families and friends providing long-term care at home. Long recognised as a pioneer in health services, FCA now offers programmes at national, state and local levels to support and sustain caregivers.
(800)-445-8106
www.caregiver.org

National Council on Aging (NCOA)
A non-profit service and advocacy organisation. A national voice for older Americans and the community organisations that serve them. Brings together non-profit organisations, businesses and government to develop creative solutions that improve the lives of all older adults.
800-677-1116
www.ncoa.org

National Institute on Aging (NIA)
The NIA – one of the 27 institutes and centers of the National Institute for Health – has been at the forefront of the Nation's research activities dedicated to understanding the nature of aging, supporting the health and well-being of older adults, and extending healthy, active years of life for more people.
1-800-222-2225
www.nia.nih.gov

Australia

Aged Care Australia
Information and support for those carrying out aged care. Aged care services in all regions.
1800 200 422
www.agedcareaustralia.gov.au

Alzheimer's Australia
Administers leading edge national dementia programmes and services funded by the Commonwealth as well as providing national policy and advocacy for the 280,000 Australians living with dementia.
1800 100 500
www.fightdementia.org.au

Australian Government Department of Health and Ageing
Better health and active ageing for all Australians.
1800 020 103
www.health.gov.au

Carers Australia
The national peak body representing Australia's 2.6 million carers. Its vision is that caring should be a shared community responsibility. Carers' support and services in all localities.
1800 242 636
www.carersaustralia.com.au

Canada

Alzheimer Society
Canada's leading health charity for people living with Alzheimer's disease and other dementias.
1-800-616-8816
www.alzheimer.ca

Canadian Dementia Action Network (CDAN)
Dedicated to eradicating Alzheimer's disease and related dementias (ADRD), CDAN brings together Canada's world-class biomedical researchers and clinicians for the purpose of quickly identifying promising treatments for ADRD.
1-604-822-7377
www.cdan.ca

New Zealand

Alzheimer's New Zealand
A support and advocacy organisation for people with dementia, their carers, family, whanau and community.
0800 004 001
www.alzheimers.org.nz

Carers New Zealand
Information and advice for family carers.
0800 777 797
www.carers.net.nz

New Zealand Ministry of Health
The government's principal adviser on health and disability: improving, promoting and protecting the health of all New Zealanders.
0800 855 066
www.health.govt.nz

Index